Ultimate Keto Air Fryer Recipe Collections

Quick and Easy Recipes For Beginners

Rudy Kent

© Copyright 2020 - All rights reserved.

The content contained within this book may not be reproduced, duplicated or transmitted without direct written permission from the author or the publisher.

Under no circumstances will any blame or legal responsibility be held against the publisher, or author, for any damages, reparation, or monetary loss due to the information contained within this book. Either directly or indirectly.

Legal Notice:

This book is copyright protected. This book is only for personal use. You cannot amend, distribute, sell, use, quote or paraphrase any part, or the content within this book, without the consent of the author or publisher.

Disclaimer Notice:

Please note the information contained within this document is for educational and entertainment purposes only. All effort has been executed to present accurate, up to date, and reliable, complete information. No warranties of any kind are declared or implied. Readers acknowledge that the author is not engaging in the rendering of legal, financial, medical or professional advice. The content within this book has been derived from various sources. Please consult a licensed professional before attempting any techniques outlined in this book.

By reading this document, the reader agrees that under no circumstances is the author responsible for any losses, direct or indirect, which are incurred as a result of the use of information contained within this document, including, but not limited to, — errors, omissions, or inaccuracies.

© **Copyright 2020 - All rights reserved.**

The content contained within this book may not be reproduced, duplicated or transmitted without direct written permission from the author or the publisher.

Under no circumstances will any blame or legal responsibility be held against the publisher, or author, for any damages, reparation, or monetary loss due to the information contained within this book. Either directly or indirectly.

Legal Notice:

This book is copyright protected. This book is only for personal use. You cannot amend, distribute, sell, use, quote or paraphrase any part, or the content within this book, without the consent of the author or publisher.

Disclaimer Notice:

Please note the information contained within this document is for educational and entertainment purposes only. All effort has been executed to present accurate, up to date, and reliable, complete information. No warranties of any kind are declared or implied. Readers acknowledge that the author is not engaging in the rendering of legal, financial, medical or professional advice. The content within this book has been derived from various sources. Please consult a licensed professional before attempting any techniques outlined in this book.

By reading this document, the reader agrees that under no circumstances is the author responsible for any losses, direct or indirect, which are incurred as a result of the use of information contained within this document, including, but not limited to, — errors, omissions, or inaccuracies.

Introduction

What's the difference between an air fryer and deep fryer? Air fryers bake food at a high temperature with a high-powered fan, while deep fryers cook food in a vat of oil that has been heated up to a specific temperature. Both cook food quickly, but an air fryer requires practically zero preheat time while a deep fryer can take upwards of 10 minutes. Air fryers also require little to no oil and deep fryers require a lot that absorb into the food. Food comes out crispy and juicy in both appliances, but don't taste the same, usually because deep fried foods are coated in batter that cook differently in an air fryer vs a deep fryer. Battered foods needs to be sprayed with oil before cooking in an air fryer to help them color and get crispy, while the hot oil soaks into the batter in a deep fryer. Flour-based batters and wet batters don't cook well in an air fryer, but they come out very well in a deep fryer.

The ketogenic diet is one such example. The diet calls for a very small number of carbs to be eaten. This means food such as rice, pasta, and other starchy vegetables like potatoes are off the menu. Even relaxed versions of the keto diet minimize carbs to a large extent and this compromises the goals of many dieters. They end up having to exert large amounts of willpower to follow the diet. This doesn't do them any favors since willpower is like a muscle. At some point, it tires and this is when the dieter goes right back to their old pattern of eating. I have personal experience with this. In terms of health benefits, the keto diet offers the most. The reduction of carbs forces your body to mobilize fat and this results in automatic fat loss and better health.

Feel free to mix and match the recipes you see in here and play around with them. Eating is supposed to be fun! Unfortunately, we've associated fun eating with unhealthy food. This doesn't have to be the case. The air fryer, combined with the Mediterranean diet, will make your mealtimes fun-filled again and full of taste. There's no grease and messy cleanups to deal with anymore. Are you excited yet?

You should be! You're about to embark on a journey full of air fried goodness!

Table of Contents

Introduction 5

Homemade Apple Chips 9
Easy and Delicious Pizza Puffs 11
Buffalo Chicken Tenders 17
Jamaican Chicken Fajitas 19
Sweet Wasabi Chicken 23
Tropical Coconut Chicken Thighs 25
Crispy Drumsticks with Blue Cheese Sauce 27
Tarragon & Garlic Roasted Chicken 30
Chicken Meatballs with Farfalle Pasta 36
Herby Chicken Schnitzels with Mozzarella 40
Air Fried Chicken Bowl with Black Beans 44
French-Style Chicken Thighs 45
Thai Chicken Satay 48
Asian Sticky Chicken Wingettes 50
Turkey Burgers with Cabbage Slaw 52
Turkey Strips with Garlic Mushrooms 54
Thai Tom Yum Wings 56
Almond-Fried Crispy Chicken 58
Chicken Quarters with Broccoli & Rice 60
Whole Chicken with Prunes 62
Rice Krispies Chicken Goujons 68
Crispy Chicken Tenders with Hot Aioli 70
Creamy Asiago Chicken 74

Creamy Onion Chicken 76

Cauli-Oat Crusted Drumsticks 78

Chicken Asian Lollipop 80

Greek-Style Chicken Wings 86

Chicken & Jalapeño Quesadilla 88

Chicken Fingers with Red Mayo Dip 90

Double Cheese Marinara Chicken 98

Chicken Thighs with Marinara Sauce 99

Whole Roasted Chicken 102

Quinoa Chicken Nuggets 104

Tex-Mex Seasoned Chicken 106

Cajun Chicken Tenders 108

Homemade Apple Chips

Cooking Time:

20 minutes

Serve: 4

Ingredients:

1 cooking apples, cored and thinly sliced
1 teaspoon peanut oil
¼ teaspoon ground cloves
¼ teaspoon ground cinnamon
1 tablespoon smooth peanut butter

Directions:

1. Toss the apple slices with the peanut oil. Bake at 350 degrees F for 5 minutes; shake the basket to ensure even cooking and continue to cook an additional 5 minutes.

2. Spread each apple slice with a little peanut butter and sprinkle with ground cloves and cinnamon. Serve and enjoy!

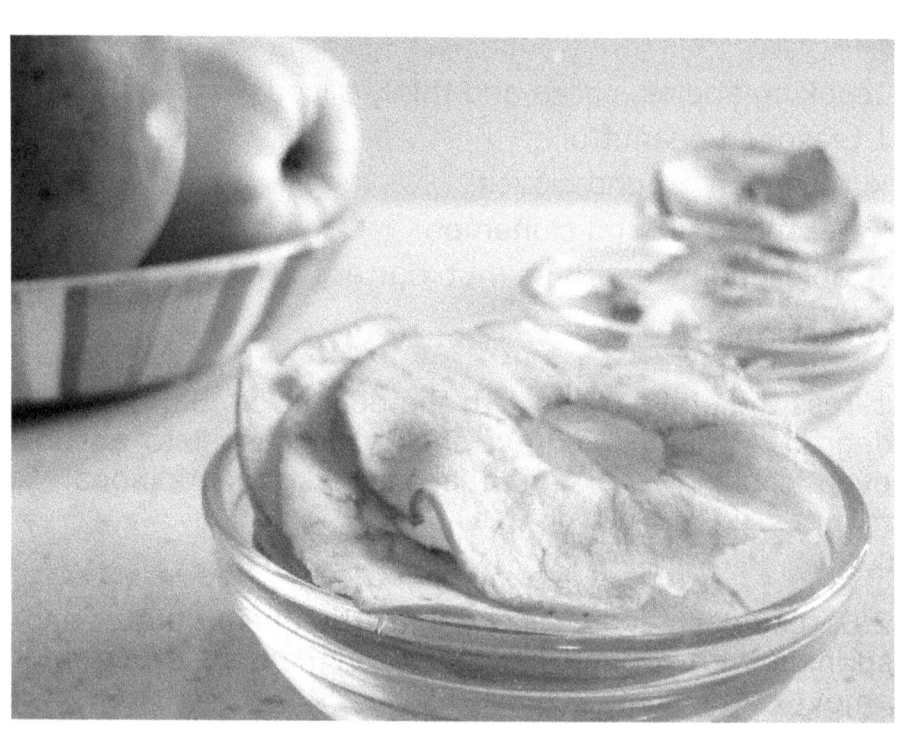

Easy and Delicious Pizza Puffs

Cooking Time:

15 minutes

Serve: 6

Ingredients:

6 ounces crescent roll dough
½ cup mozzarella cheese, shredded
3 ounces pepperoni
3 ounces mushrooms, chopped
1 teaspoon oregano
1 teaspoon garlic powder
¼ cup Marina sauce, for dipping

Directions:

1. Unroll the crescent dough. Roll out the dough using a rolling pin; cut into 6 pieces.

2. Place the cheese, pepperoni, and mushrooms in the center of each pizza puff. Sprinkle with oregano and garlic powder.

3. Fold each corner over the filling using wet hands. Press together to cover the filling entirely and seal the edges.

4. Now, spritz the bottom of the Air Fryer basket with cooking oil. Lay the pizza puffs in a single layer in the cooking basket. Work in batches. Bake at 370 degrees

F for 5 to 6 minutes or until golden brown.
5.Serve with the marinara sauce for dipping.

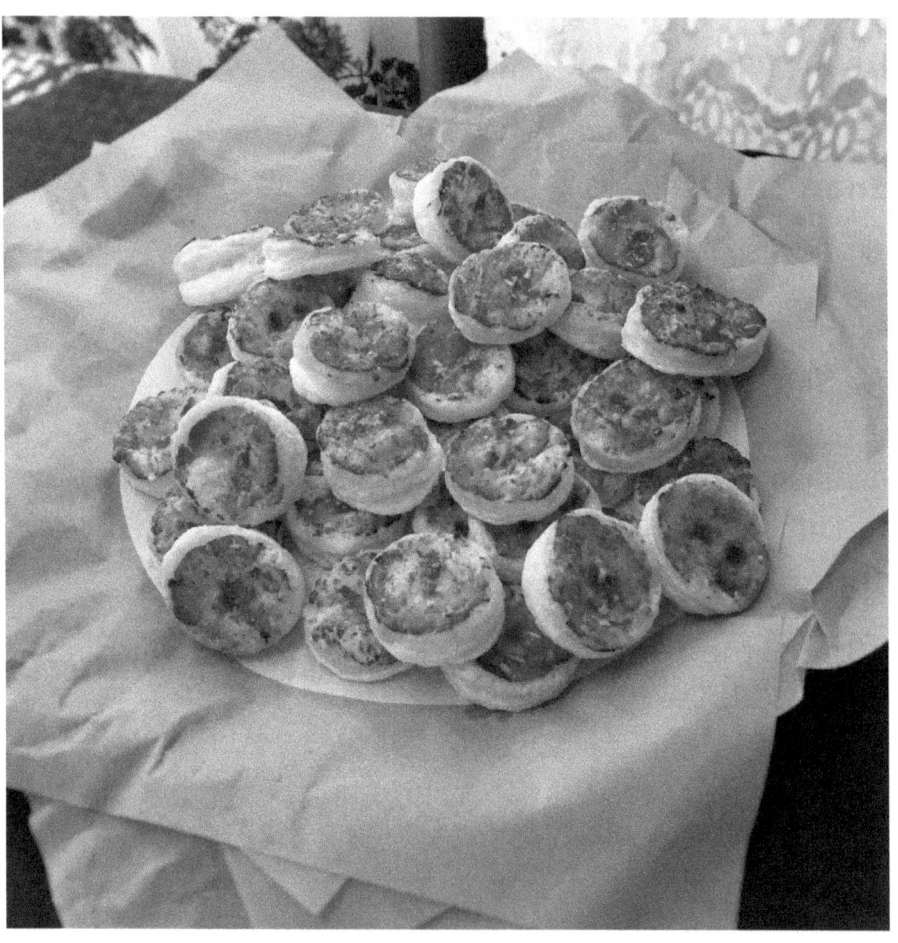

Party Greek Keftedes

Cooking Time:

20 minutes

Serve: 6

Ingredients:

Greek Keftedes:

½ pound mushrooms, chopped
½ pound pork sausage, chopped
1 teaspoon shallot powder
1 teaspoon granulated garlic
1 teaspoon dried rosemary
1 teaspoon dried basil
1 teaspoon dried oregano
2 eggs
2 tablespoons cornbread crumbs

Tzatziki Dip:

1 Lebanese cucumbers, grated, juice squeezed out 1 cup full-fat Greek yogurt

1 tablespoon fresh lemon juice

1 garlic clove, minced

1 tablespoon extra-virgin olive oil

½ teaspoon salt

Directions:

1. In a mixing bowl, thoroughly combine all ingredients for the Greek keftedes. Shape the meat mixture into bite-sized balls.

2.Cook in the preheated Air Fryer at 380 degrees for 10 minutes, shaking the cooking basket once or twice to ensure even cooking.

3.Meanwhile, make the tzatziki dip by mixing all ingredients. Serve the keftedes with cocktail sticks and tzatziki dip on the side. Enjoy!

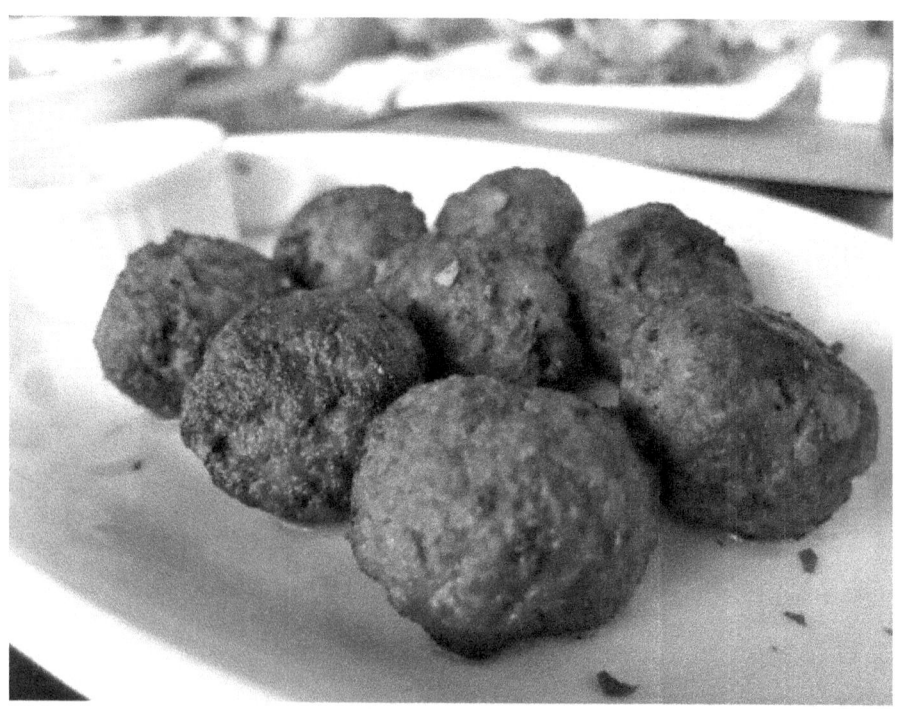

South Asian Chicken Strips

Cooking Time:

35 minutes

Serve:4

Ingredients:

1 lb chicken breasts, cut into strips
2 tomatoes, cubed
1 green chili pepper, cut into stripes
½ tsp cumin
2 green onions, sliced
2 tbsp olive oil
1 tbsp yellow mustard
½ tsp ginger powder
2 tbsp fresh cilantro, chopped
Salt and black pepper to taste

Directions:

1. Heat olive oil in a deep pan over medium heat and sauté mustard, green onions, ginger powder, cumin, and green chili pepper for 2-3 minutes.

2. Stir in tomatoes, cilantro, and salt; set aside. Preheat the air fryer to 380 F. Season the chicken with salt and pepper, and place in the greased air fryer basket. Air Fry for 15 minutes, shaking once.

3. Top with the sauce and serve.

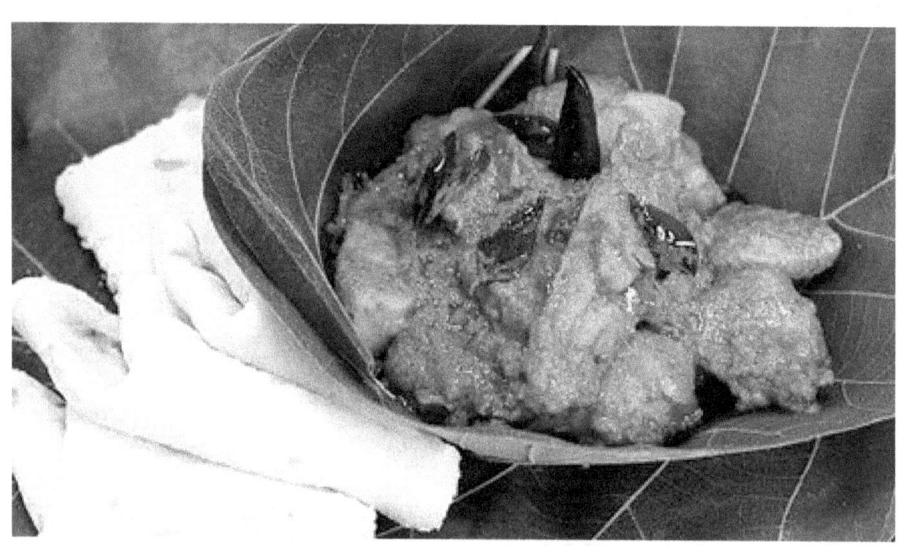

Buffalo Chicken Tenders

Cooking Time:

25 minutes

Serve: 4

Ingredients:

1 cup breadcrumbs
½ cup yogurt
1 lb chicken breasts, cut into strips
½ tsp red chili pepper
1 tbsp hot sauce
2 eggs, beaten
1 tsp sweet paprika
1 tsp garlic powder

Directions:

1. Preheat air fryer to 390 F. Whisk eggs with the hot sauce and yogurt. In a shallow bowl, combine the breadcrumbs, paprika, cayenne pepper, and garlic powder.

2. Line a baking dish with parchment paper. Dip the chicken in the egg/yogurt mixture first, and then coat with breadcrumbs.

3. Arrange on the sheet and Bake in the air fryer for 8-10 minutes. Flip the chicken over and bake for 6-8 more minutes. Serve.

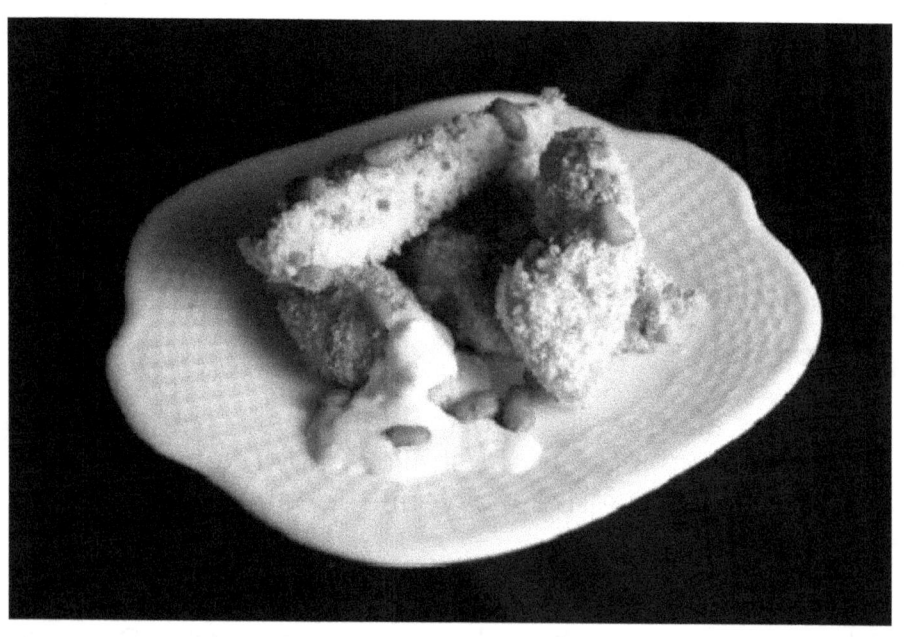

Jamaican Chicken Fajitas

Cook Time:

25minutes

Servings: 4

Ingredients:

1 lb chicken tenderloins
1 cup Jamaican jerk seasoning
2 tbsp lime juice
2 tbsp olive oil
4 large tortilla wraps
1 cup julienned carrots
1 cucumber, peeled, sliced
1 cup shredded lettuce
1 cup coleslaw mix
½ cup mango chutney

Directions:

1. Whisk the olive oil, jerk seasoning, and lime juice in a bowl. Add in the chicken and toss to coat. Put in the fridge for 1 hour.

2. Remove the chicken from the fridge, keeping the leftover marinade to the side. Preheat air fryer to 380 F.

3. Arrange the chicken tenderloins on the greased fryer basket in a single layer. Air Fry for 8 minutes. Flip the chicken and brush with more marinade. Fry for 5-7 more minutes.

4. Divide the coleslaw mix carrots, cucumber, lettuce, and mango chutney between the tortillas. Add the chicken tenderloins on top and roll up the tortillas. Serve warm or cold.

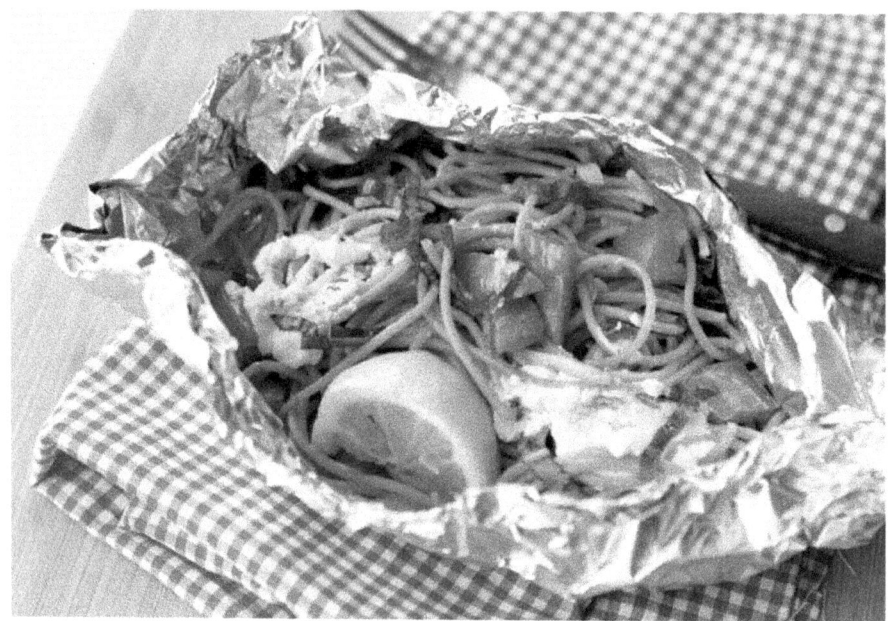

Easy Chicken Enchiladas

Cooking Time:

40 minutes

Serve: 4

Ingredients:

1lb chicken breasts, chopped
1 cup mozzarella cheese, grated
½ cup salsa
1 can green chilies, chopped
8 flour tortillas
1 cup enchilada sauce

Directions:

1. Preheat the air fryer to 400 F. In a bowl, mix salsa and enchilada sauce.

2. Toss in the chopped chicken to coat. Place the chicken in a baking dish and Bake in the air fryer for 14-18 minutes, shaking once. Remove and divide between the tortillas.

3. Top with cheese and roll the tortillas. Place in the air fryer basket and Bake for 10 minutes. Serve with guacamole.

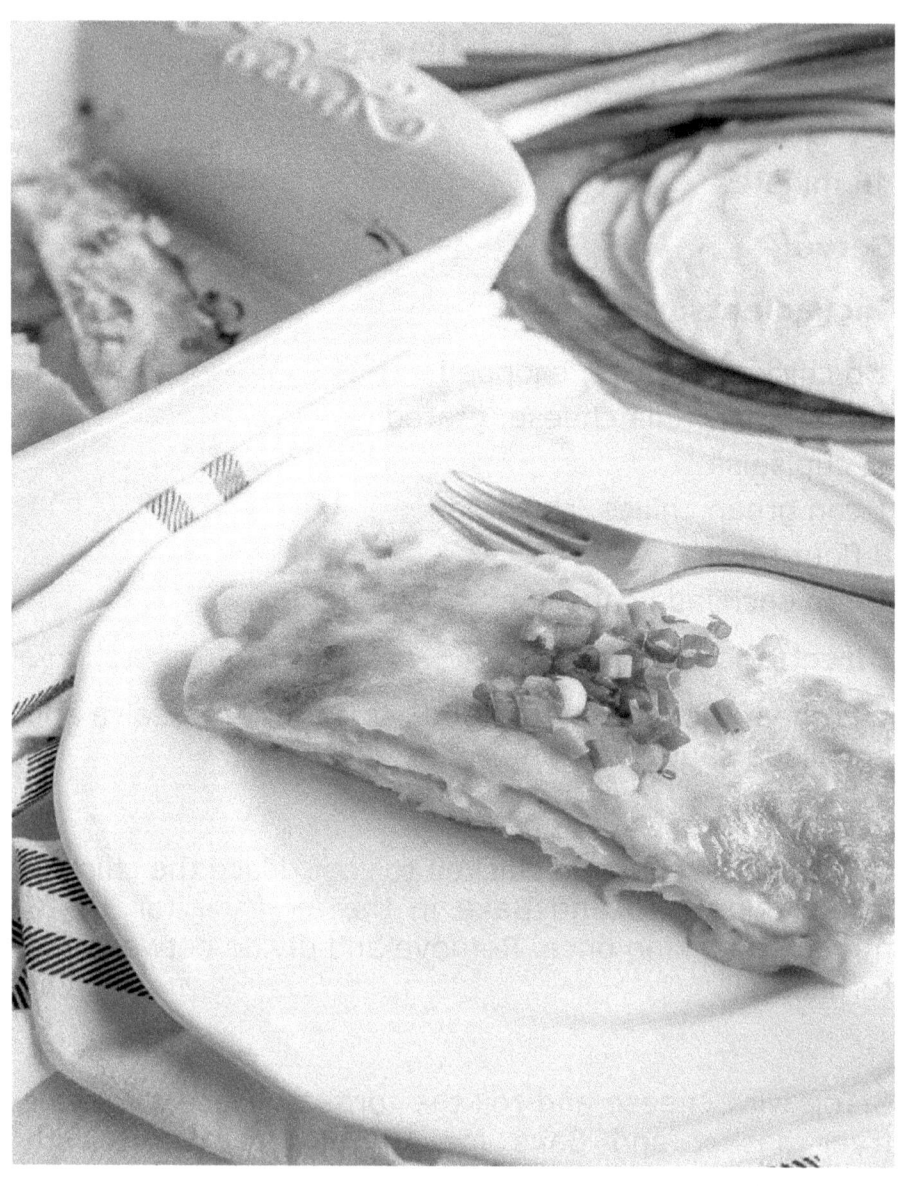

Sweet Wasabi Chicken

Cooking Time:

20 minutes

Serve: 4

Iingredients:

1tbsp wasabi

1 tbsp agave syrup

2 tsp black sesame seeds

Salt and black pepper to taste

2 chicken breasts, cut into larg chunks

Directions:

1.In a bowl, mix wasabi, agave syrup, sesame seed, salt, and pepper.

2.Rub the mixture onto the breasts. Arrange the breasts on a greased frying basket and cook for 16 minutes, turning once halfway through.

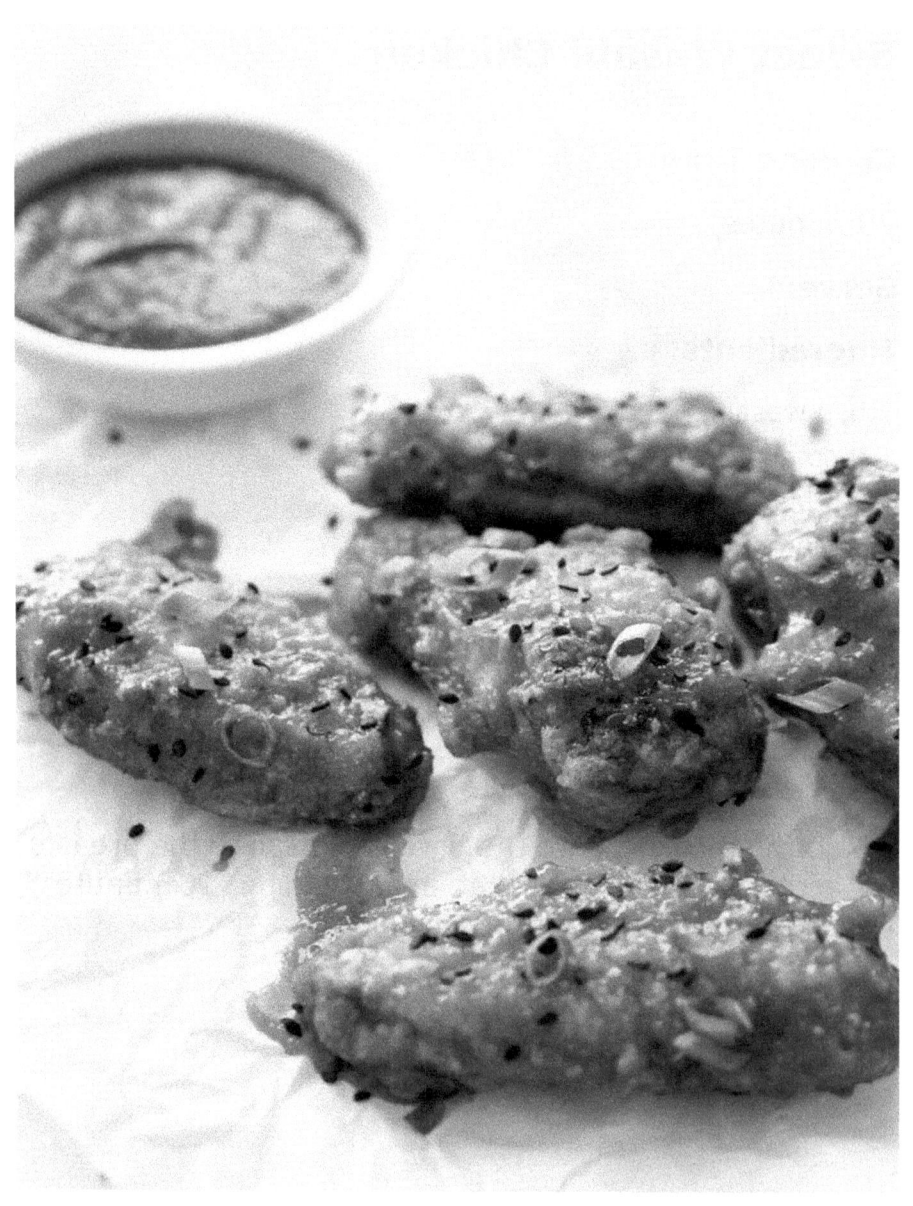

Tropical Coconut Chicken Thighs

Cooking Time:

20 minutes

Serve: 4

Ingredients:

1 tbsp curry powder
4 tbsp mango chutney
Salt and black pepper to taste
¾ cup coconut, shredded
1 lb chicken thighs

Directions:

1. Preheat air fryer to 400 F. In a bowl, mix curry powder, mango chutney, salt, and black pepper.

2. Brush the thighs with the glaze and roll the chicken thighs in shredded coconut.

3. Grease a baking dish with cooking spray and arrange the thing in. Bake them in the air fryer for 12-14 minutes, turning once, until golden brown.

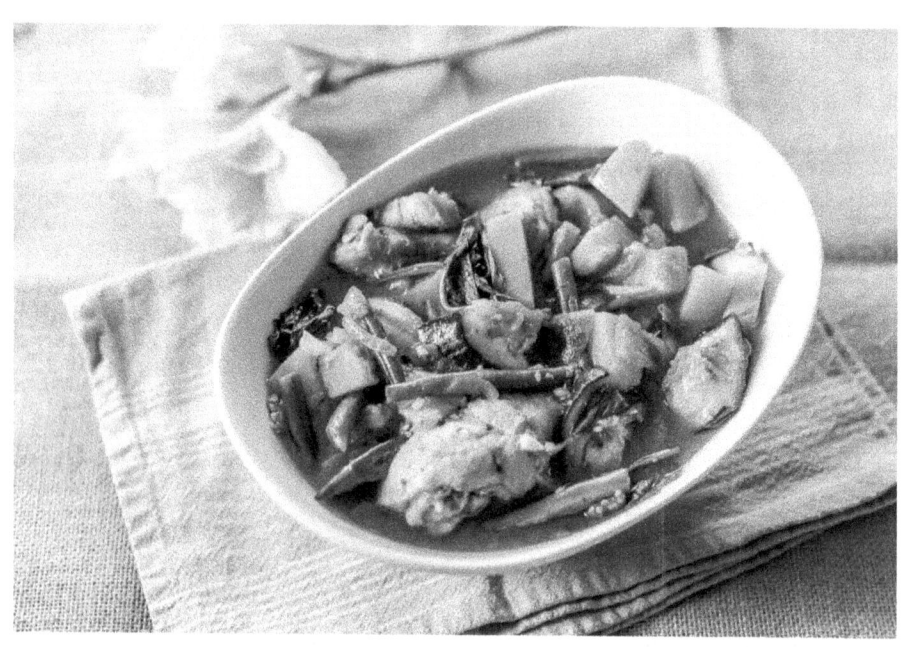

Crispy Drumsticks with Blue Cheese Sauce

Cooking Time:

30 minutes

Serve: 4

Ingredients:

Drumsticks:
1 lb drumsticks
3 tbsp butter
1 tsp paprika
¼ cup hot sauce
1 tsp onion powder
1 tsp garlic powder

Blue Cheese Sauce:

½ cup mayonnaise

1 cup blue cheese, crumbled

1 cup sour cream

½ tsp garlic powder

½ tsp onion powder

Salt and black pepper to taste

½ tsp cayenne pepper

1 ½ tsp white wine vinegar

2 tbsp buttermilk

1 ½ tsp Worcestershire sauce

Directions:

1. Melt the butter in a skillet over medium heat and stir in the remaining drumstick ingredients, except for the drumsticks.

2. Cook the mixture for 5 minutes or until the sauce reduces; then let cool.

3. Place the drumsticks in a bowl, pour the cooled sauce over, and coat well. Refrigerate for 2 hours.

4. In a jug, add sour cream, blue cheese, mayonnaise, garlic powder, onion powder, buttermilk, cayenne pepper, white wine vinegar, Worcestershire sauce, black pepper, and salt.

5. Using a stick mixer, blend the ingredients until well mixed with no large lumps. Adjust the seasoning. Preheat air fryer to 350 F.

6. Remove the drumsticks from the fridge and place them in the frying basket to Bake for 15 minutes. Turn the drumsticks with tongs every 5 minutes to ensure they cook evenly.

7. Serve with blue cheese sauce and a side of celery sticks.

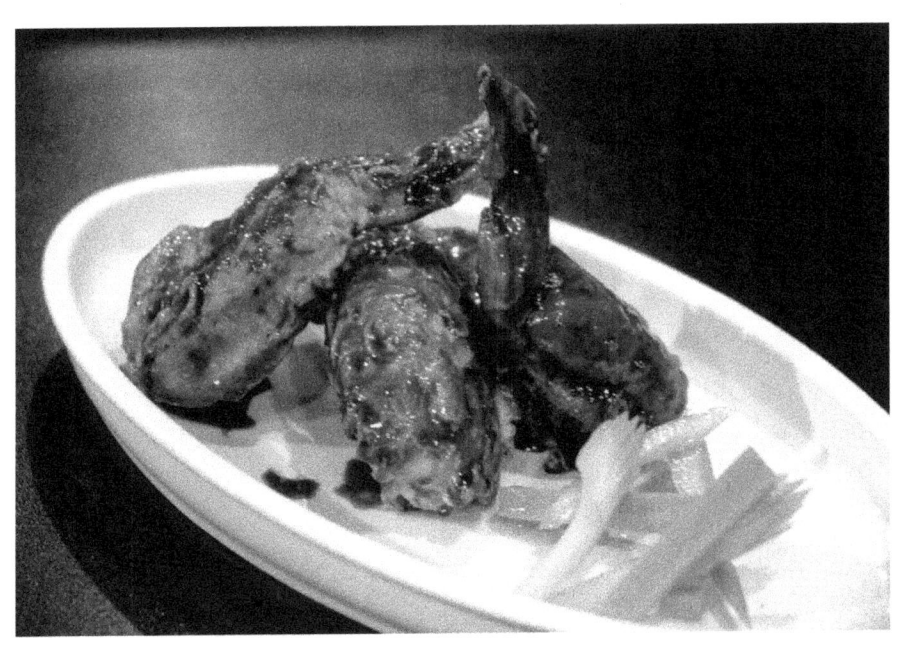

Tarragon & Garlic Roasted Chicken

Cooking Time:

50 minutes

Serve: 4

Ingredients:

1 chicken around
3 lb 1 tsp fresh tarragon, chopped
2 tbsp butter, melted
Salt and black pepper to taste
1 lemon, cut into wedges
1 garlic bulb

Directions:

1. Preheat air fryer to 380 F. Brush the chicken with melted butter and season with salt and pepper. Put tarragon, garlic, and lemon into the cavity of the chicken and place in the air fryer basket.

2. Bake for 40 minutes. Cover with foil and let rest for 10 minutes, then carve, and serve with fresh salad.

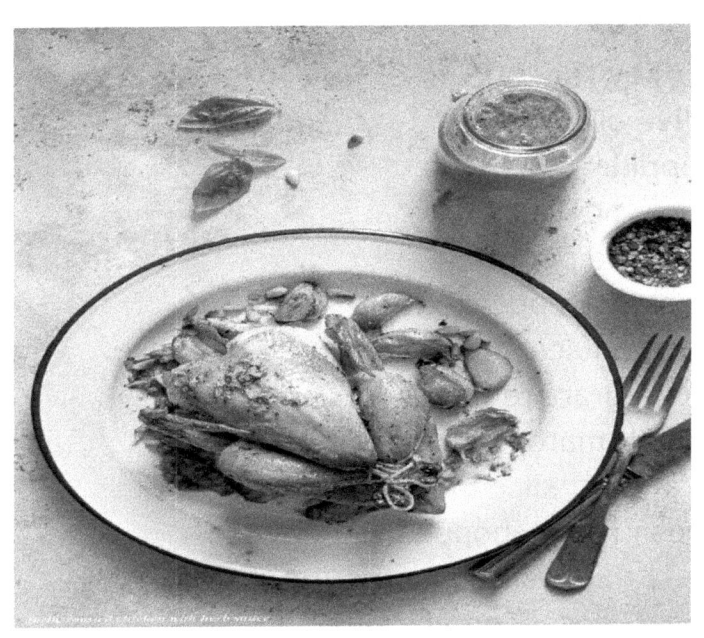

Turkey Tenderloins with Fattoush Salad

Cooking Time:

50 minutes

Serve: 4

Ingredients:

1 ½ lb turkey tenderloins
3 tbsp olive oil
½ tsp paprika
½ tsp garlic powder
½ tsp cayenne pepper
Salt and black pepper to taste
1 tbsp lemon juice
1 tbsp pomegranate molasses
½ lb Roma tomatoes, chopped
2 spring onions, sliced
2 tbsp fresh mint, chopped
6 radishes, thinly sliced
1 cucumber, deseeded and diced
5 oz pita crackers

Directions:

1. In a bowl, mix the lemon juice, 2 tbsp of the olive oil, pomegranate molasses, and salt and whisk with a fork.

2. Add in the tomatoes, spring onions, radishes, cucumber, fresh mint and toss to coat. Reserve. Preheat your Air Fryer to 375°F.

3.Combine the paprika, garlic powder, salt, black pepper, and cayenne pepper in a small bowl, then rub the mixture all over the turkey.

4.Put the turkey in the greased fryer basket and spray with olive oil, then air fry for 15 minutes. Turn it over and spray it again, then cook for 10-15 more minutes.

5.Remove the turkey and let it sit for 5-8 minutes before slicing. Transfer the salad to a serving dish and top with pita crackers. Serve the turkey with the salad and enjoy!

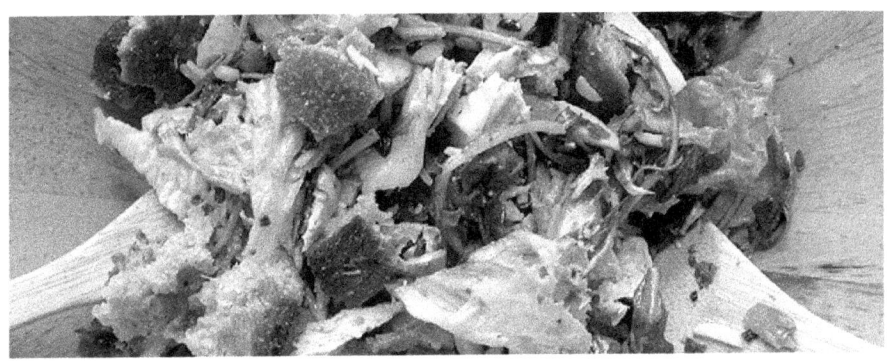

Sweet Chili & Ginger Chicken Wings

Cooking Time:

20 minutes

Serve: 4

Ingredients:

1 lb chicken wings
1 tsp ginger root powder
1 tbsp tamarind powder
¼ cup sweet chili sauce

Directions:

1. Preheat air fryer to 390 F. Rub the chicken wings with tamarind and ginger root powders. Spray with cooking spray and place in the air fryer basket.

2. Cook for 6 minutes. Slide-out the basket and cover with sweet chili sauce; cook for 8 more minutes. Serve warm.

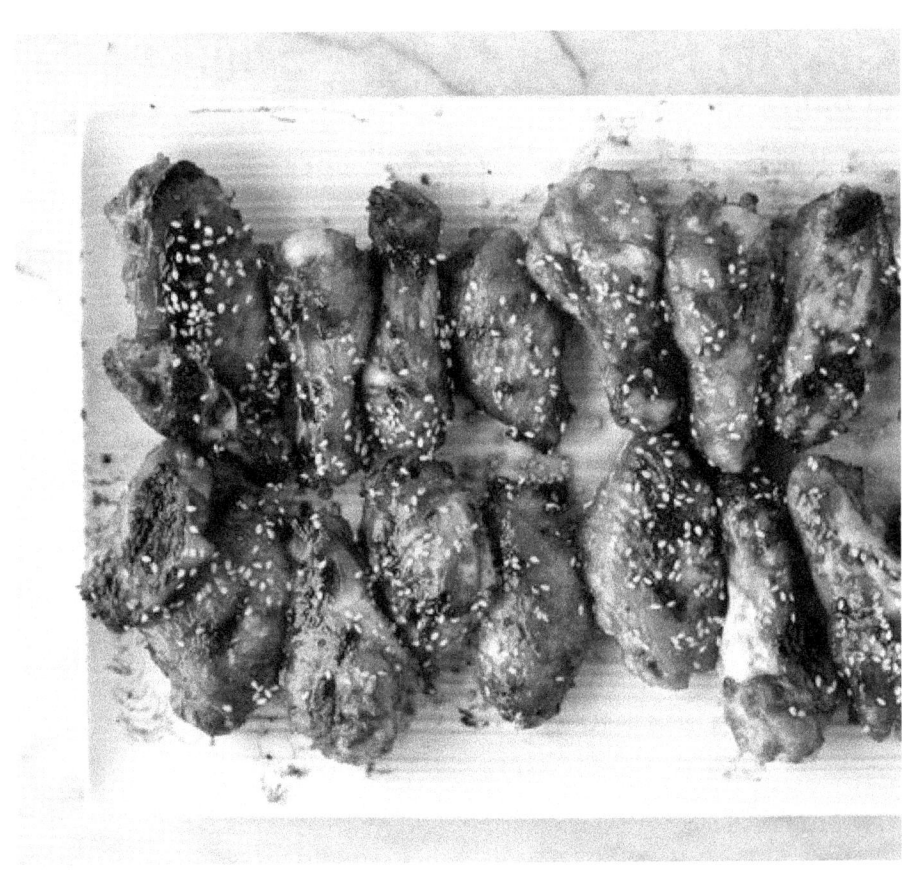

Chicken Meatballs with Farfalle Pasta
Cooking Time:

50 minutes

Serve: 6

Ingredients:

1lb ground chicken
3 tbsp olive oil
4 oz fresh spinach, chopped
½ cup panko bread crumbs
¼ tsp garlic powder
1 egg, beaten
⅓ cup feta cheese, crumbled
8 oz farfalle pasta, cooked
2 cups marinara sauce
Salt and black pepper to taste

Directions:

1. Preheat air fryer to 360 F. Warm 2 tbsp of the olive oil in a large skillet over medium heat and add the spinach.

2. Season with salt and cook for 2-3 minutes or until the spinach has wilted. Set aside.

3. Mix the panko breadcrumbs, salt, pepper, and garlic powder in a bowl. Add the egg, ground chicken, spinach, and feta and stir to combine.

4. Shape the mixture into 1-inch balls. Arrange them in a single layer on the greased fryer basket and spray with the remaining olive oil.

5.Air fry for 7 minutes, shake them, and cook another 5-8 minutes or until golden. Serve the chicken meatballs on farfalle pasta and spoon over the marinara sauce. Enjoy!

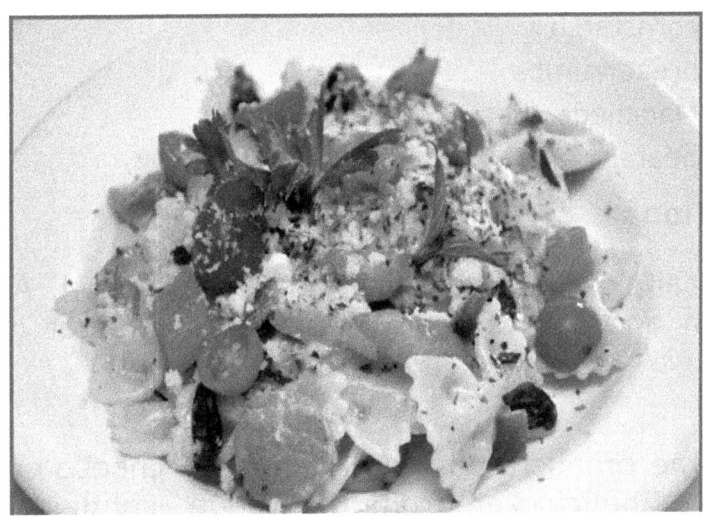

Spanish-Style Crusted Chicken Fingers

Cooking Time:

25 minutes

Serve: 2

Ingredients:

1 chicken breasts, cut into strips
Salt and black pepper to taste
1 tsp garlic powder
3 tbsp cornstarch
4 tbsp breadcrumbs
4 tbsp Manchego cheese, grated
1 egg, beaten

Directions:

1. Mix salt, garlic, and black pepper in a bowl. Add in chicken and stir to coat. Marinate for 1 hour in the fridge.

2. Mix the breadcrumbs with Manchego cheese evenly. Remove the chicken from the fridge, lightly toss in cornstarch, dip in egg and coat them gently in the cheese mixture.

3. Preheat air fryer to 350 F. Place the chicken in the greased frying basket and Bake for 15 minutes, shaking once until nice and crispy. Serve with a side of vegetable fries. Yummy!

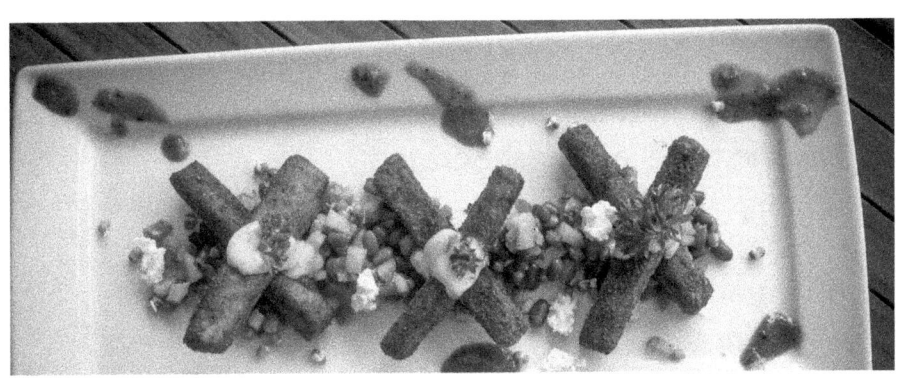

Herby Chicken Schnitzels with Mozzarella

Cooking Time:

25 minutes

Serve: 2

Ingredients:

2 chicken breasts
2 eggs, beaten
4 tbsp tomato sauce
2 tbsp mixed herbs
2 cups mozzarella cheese, grated
1 cup flour
¾ cup ham, shaved
1 cup breadcrumbs

Directions:

1. Flatten out each piece of the chicken breast using a rolling pin Place the chicken between 2 plastic sheets; flatten out it using a rolling pin.

2. Place the eggs, flour, and crumbs in 3 different bowls. Coat the chicken in the flour, followed by the eggs, and finally the crumbs.

3. Preheat air fryer to 350 F. Put the chicken in the greased frying basket and Air Fry for 10 minutes. Remove them to a plate and top with ham, tomato sauce, mozzarella cheese, and mixed herbs. Return to the fryer and AirFry further for 5 minutes or until the

mozzarella cheese melts. Serve warm.

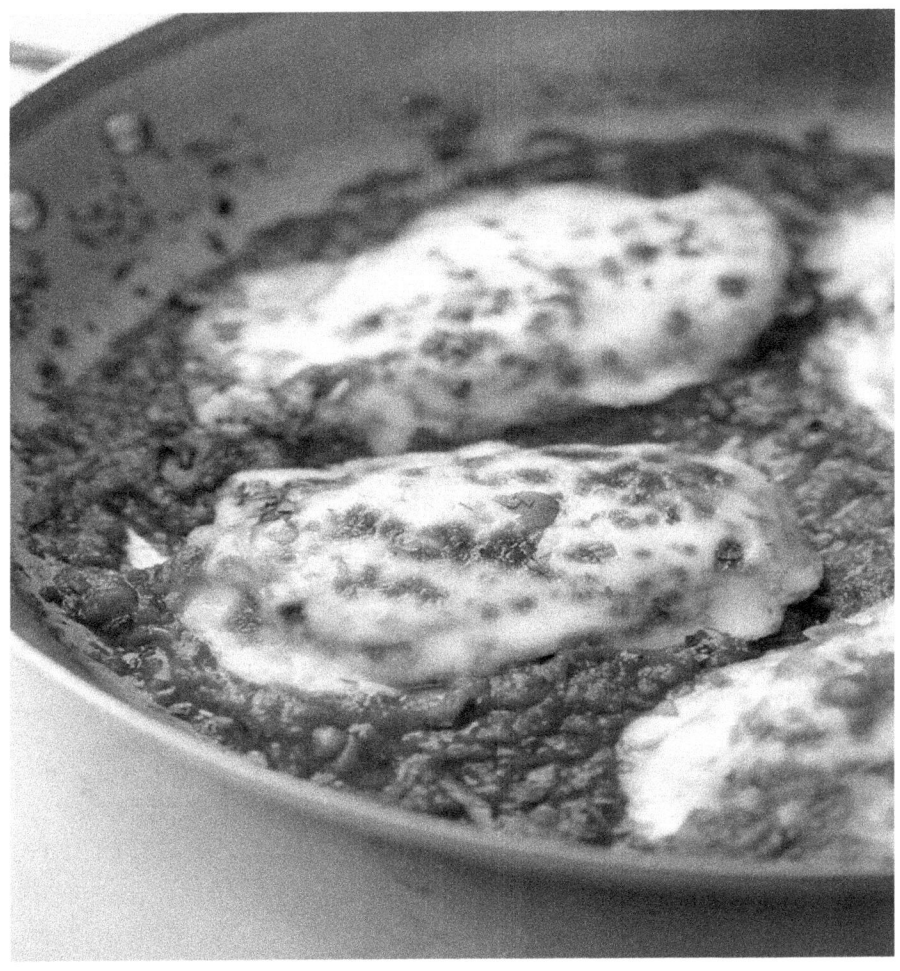

Prosciutto-Wrapped Chicken Breasts

Cooking Time:

25 minutes

Serve: 2

Ingredients:

2 chicken breasts

1 tbsp olive oil

Salt and black pepper to taste

1 cup semi-dried tomatoes, sliced

2 brie cheese slices

4 thin prosciutto slices

Directions:

1. Preheat air fryer to 370 F. Put the chicken breasts on a chopping board and cut a small incision deep enough to make stuffing possible.

2. Insert 1 slice of brie cheese and 4-5 tomato slices into each cut. Lay the prosciutto on the chopping board.

3. Put the chicken on one side and roll the prosciutto over the breast, making sure that both ends of the prosciutto meet under the chicken.

4. Drizzle with olive oil and sprinkle with salt and pepper. Place the chicken in the frying basket and Bake for 14-16 minutes, turning once halfway through. Slice each chicken breast in half and serve.

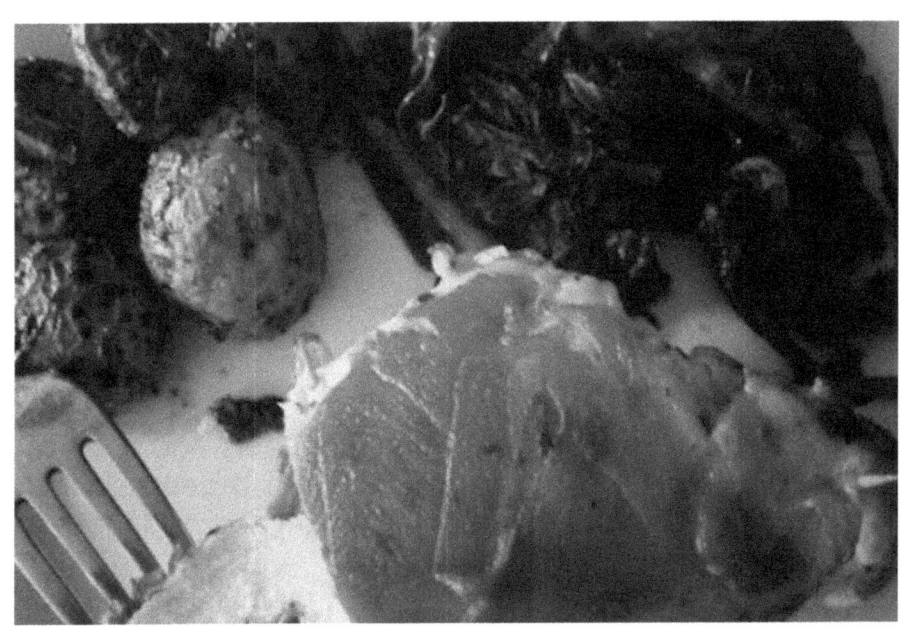

Air Fried Chicken Bowl with Black Beans

Cooking Time:

18 minutes

Serve: 4

Ingredients:

4 chicken breasts, cubed
1 can sweet corn
1 can black beans, rinsed and drained
1 cup red and green peppers, stripes, cooked
1 tbsp vegetable oil
1 tsp chili powder

Directions:

1. Coat the chicken with salt, black pepper, and a bit of oil. Air Fry for 15 minutes at 380 F. In a deep skillet, pour 1 tbsp of oil and stir in chili powder, corn, peppers, and beans.

2. Add a little bit of hot water and keep stirring for 3 minutes. Transfer the veggies to a serving platter and top with the fried chicken.

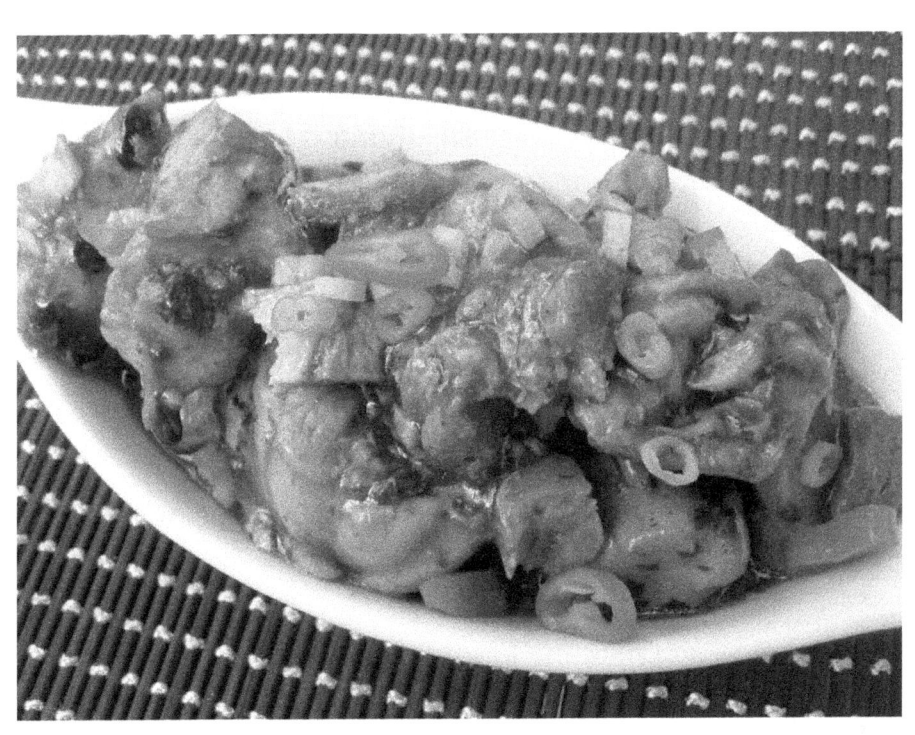

French-Style Chicken Thighs

Cooking Time:

20 minutes

Serve: 4

Ingredients:

1 tbsp herbs de Provence
1 lb bone-in, skinless chicken thighs
Salt and black pepper to taste
2 garlic cloves, minced
½ cup honey
¼ cup Dijon mustard
2 tbsp butter
2 tbsp fresh dill, chopped

Directions:

1. Preheat air fryer to 390 F. In a bowl, mix herbes de Provence, salt, and pepper.

2. Rub onto the chicken. Transfer to the greased air fryer basket and Bake for 15 minutes, flipping once halfway through.

3. Melt butter in a saucepan over medium heat. Stir in honey, mustard, and garlic; cook until reduced to a thick consistency, about 3 minutes. Serve the chicken drizzled with the honey-mustard sauce.

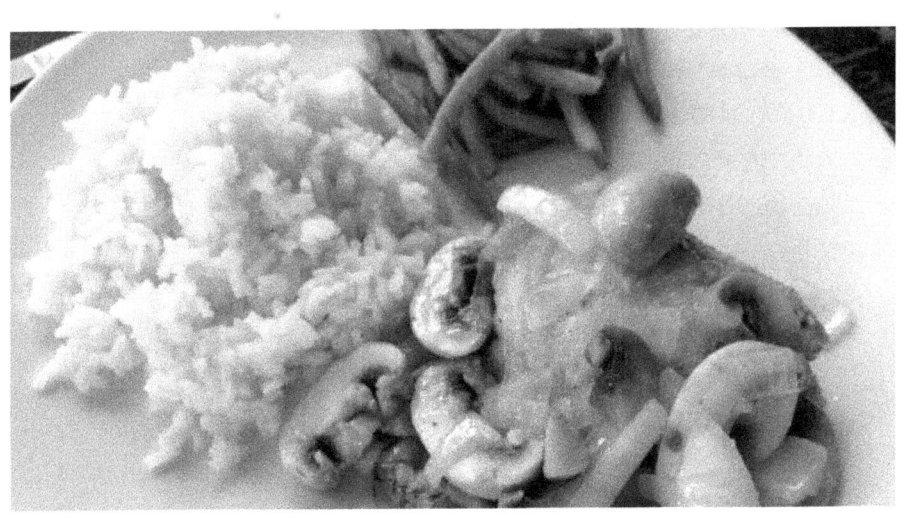

Thai Chicken Satay

Cooking Time:

25 minute

Serve: 4

Ingredients:

1 lb chicken drumsticks
2 cloves garlic, minced
2 tbsp sesame oil
½ cup Thai peanut satay sauce
1 lime, zested and juiced
2 tbsp sesame seeds, toasted
4 scallions, chopped 1 red chili, sliced

Directions:

1. In a bowl, mix the satay sauce, sesame oil, garlic, lime zest, and juice.

2. Add in the chicken and toss to coat. Place in the fridge for 2 hours to marinate. Preheat air fryer to 380 F. Transfer the marinated chicken to the frying basket and Air Fry for 18-20 minutes, flipping once halfway through.

3. Garnish with sesame seeds, scallions, and red chili and serve.

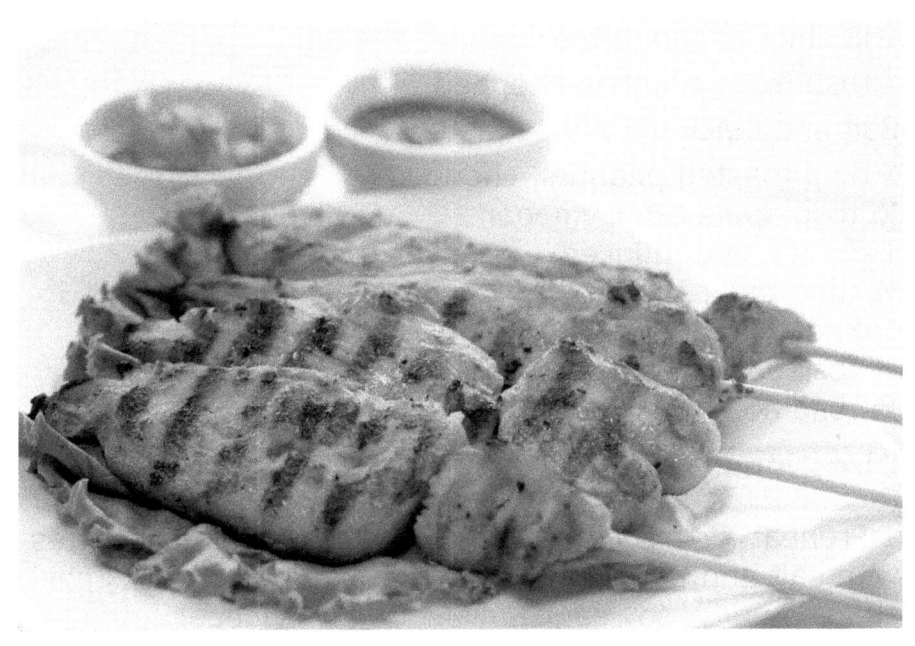

Asian Sticky Chicken Wingettes

Cooking Time:

25 minutes

Serve: 4

Ingredients:

1 lb chicken wingettes
1 tbsp fresh cilantro, chopped
Salt and black pepper to taste
1 tbsp roasted peanuts, chopped
½ tbsp apple cider vinegar
1 garlic clove, minced
½ tbsp chili sauce
1 ginger, minced 1
½ tbsp soy sauce
½ tbsp honey

Directions:

1. Preheat air fryer to 360 F. Season chicken wingettes with salt and pepper. In a bowl, mix ginger, garlic, chili sauce, honey, soy sauce, cilantro, and vinegar.

2. Cover chicken with the mixture. Transfer to the air fryer basket and cook for 14-16 minutes, shaking once. Serve sprinkled with peanuts.

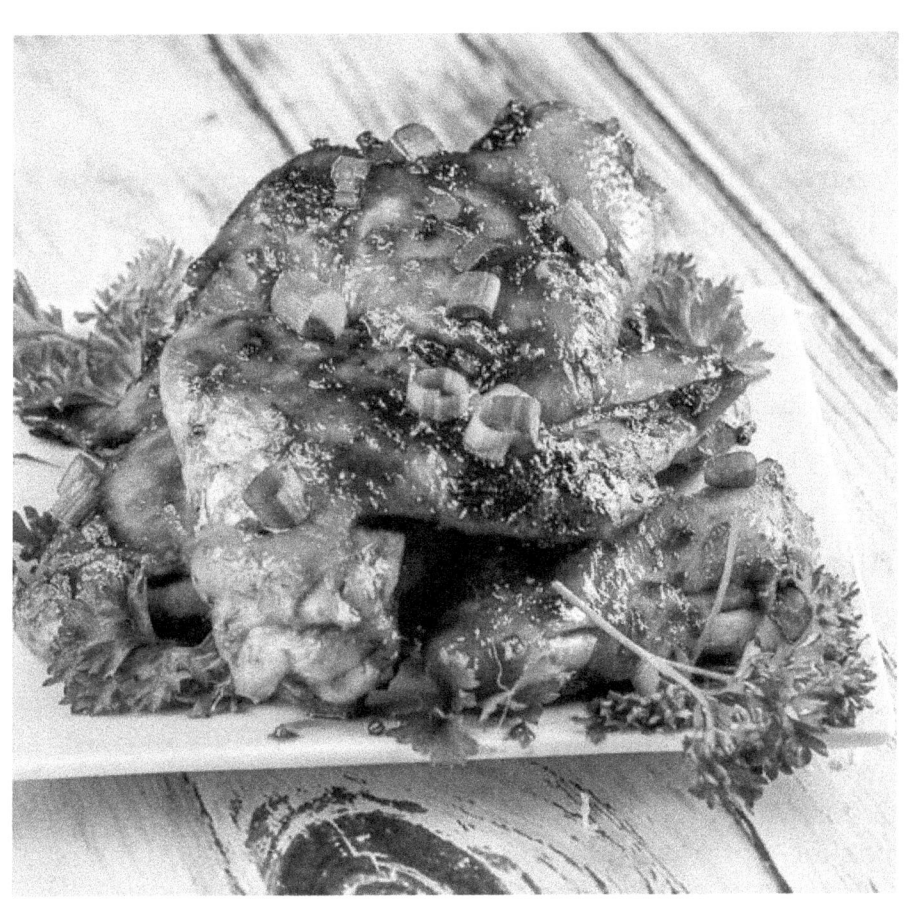

Turkey Burgers with Cabbage Slaw

Cooking Time:

60 minutes

Serve: 4

Ingredients:

1lb ground turkey

¼ cup bread crumbs

1 tbsp olive oil

¼ cup hoisin sauce

4 buns

2 green onions, slice

1 cup cabbage slaw

1 cup cherry tomatoes, halved

Directions:

1. Preheat air fryer to 375°F. Mix the turkey, breadcrumbs, and hoisin sauce in a bowl and create 4 equal patties.

2. Put the patties in a single layer in the greased fryer basket, spray with olive oil, and air fry for 10 minutes.

3. Turn the patties, spray with oil again, and cook for 5-10 more minutes or until golden. Put the burgers on buns and top with cherry tomatoes, green onions, and cabbage slaw. Serve and enjoy!

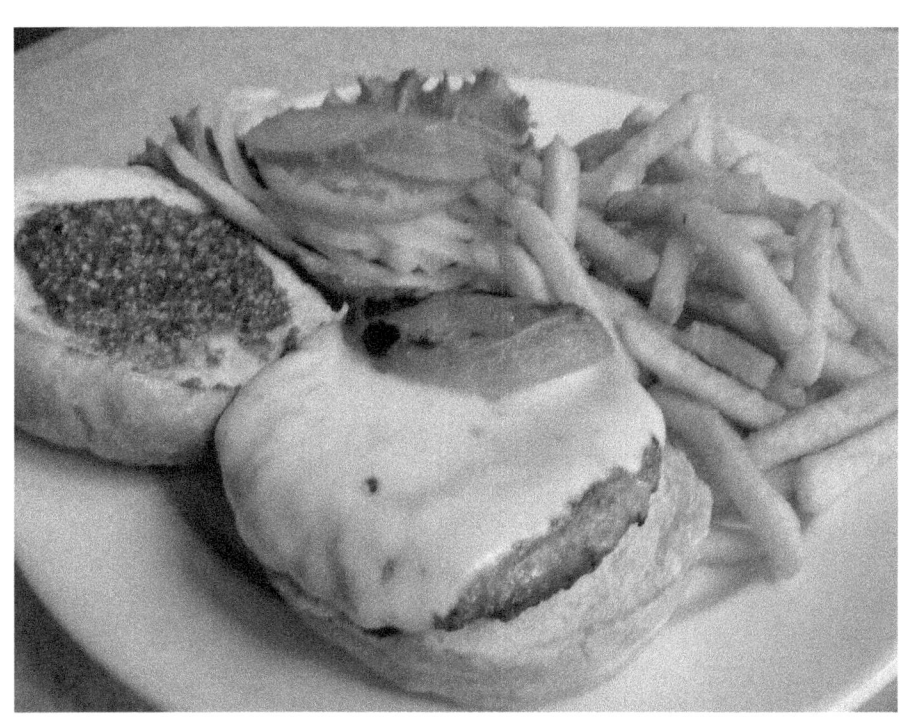

Turkey Strips with Garlic Mushrooms

Cooking Time:

20 minutes

Serve: 4

Ingredients:

1lb portobello mushrooms, sliced
1 lb turkey breast strips
½ tsp garlic powder
2 tbsp olive oil
2 tsp herbs
Salt and black pepper to taste

Directions:

1. In a bowl, mix turkey, mushrooms, olive oil, garlic powder, salt, pepper, and herbs and pour in vermouth.

2. Mix to coat. Let marinate for 15 minutes. Preheat air fryer to 350 F. Place the turkey and mushrooms in a greased baking dish and Bake for 13-15 minutes, shaking once. Serve warm.

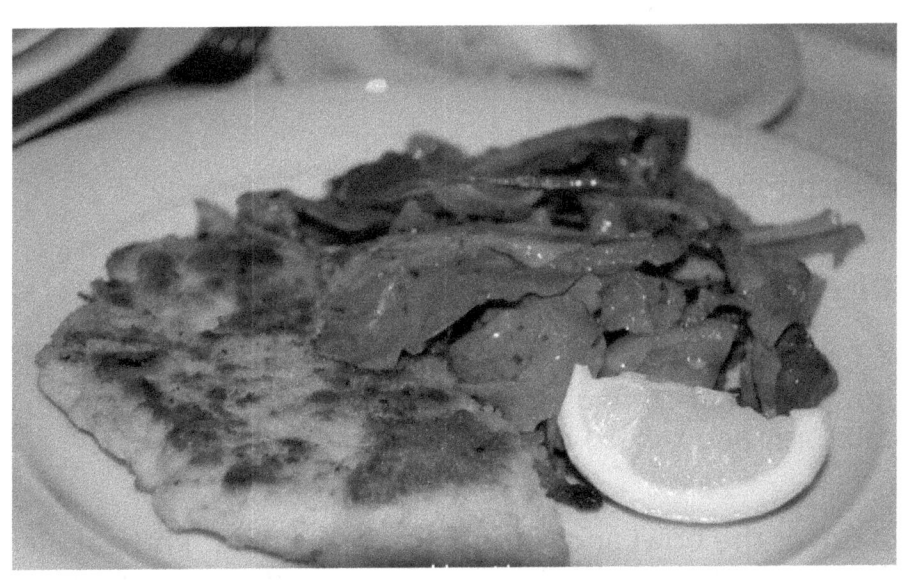

Thai Tom Yum Wings

Cooking Time:

20 minutes

Serve: 2

Ingredients:

8 chicken wings
1 tbsp water
½ cup flour
2 tbsp cornstarch
2 tbsp tom yum paste
½ tbsp baking powder

Directions:

1. Combine the tom yum paste and water in a small bowl. Place the wings in a large bowl, add the tom yum mixture, and mix to coat well.

2. Cover the bowl and refrigerate for 2 hours. Preheat air fryer to 370 F. Mix baking powder, cornstarch, and flour.

3. Dip the wings in the starch mixture. Place on the greased frying basket and Air Fry for 7-8 minutes. Flip and cook for 5-6 minutes. Serve.

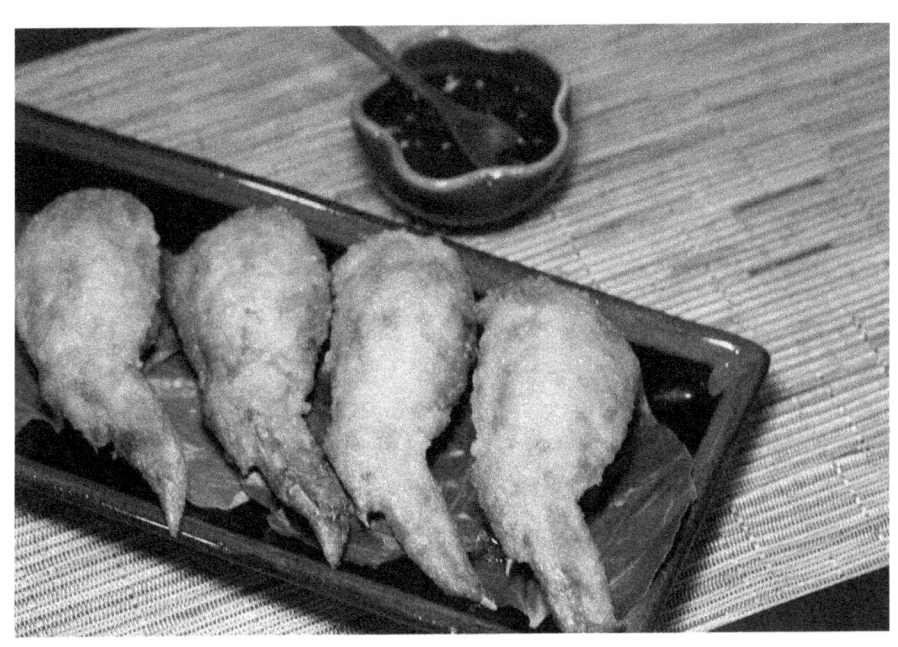

Almond-Fried Crispy Chicken

Cooking Time:

20 minutes

Serve: 4

Ingredients:

4 chicken breasts, cubed
2 cups almond meal
3 whole eggs
½ cup cornstarch
Salt and black pepper to taste
1 tbsp cayenne pepper

Directions:

1. Preheat air fryer to 350 F. In a bowl, mix salt, pepper, cornstarch, and cayenne pepper and coat the chicken.

2. In another bowl, beat the eggs. In a third bowl, pour almond meal.

3. Dredge chicken in the egg, then in almond meal, and place in the greased frying basket. Air Fry for 14-16 minutes, shaking once.

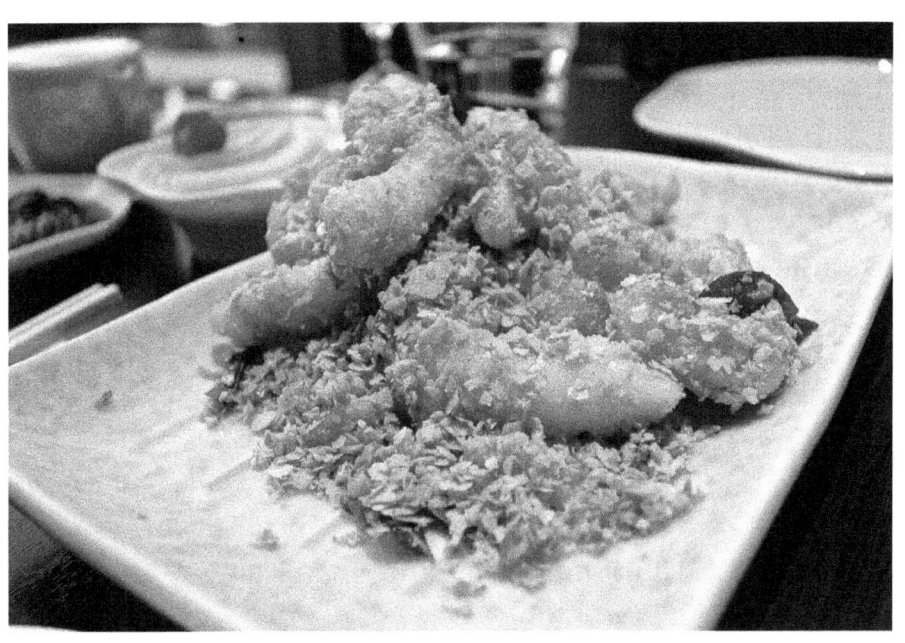

Chicken Quarters with Broccoli & Rice

Cooking Time:

30 minutes

Serve: 4

Ingredients:

4 chicken legs
1 cup long-grain rice
1 cup broccoli florets, chopped
Salt and black pepper to taste
1 can condensed cream chicken soup
1 garlic clove, minced

Directions:

1. Preheat air fryer to 390 F. Season the chicken with salt and pepper and place in the greased air fryer basket.

2. Air Fry for 10 minutes, flipping once halfway through. Place a pot over medium heat and pour in the rice, 1 cup of water, garlic, and chicken soup; bring to a boil.

3. Reduce the heat and simmer for 10 minutes. Fluff with a fork and add in broccoli. Spread the rice mixture on the bottom of a baking dish and top with chicken. Put in the air fryer and Bake for 5 minutes.

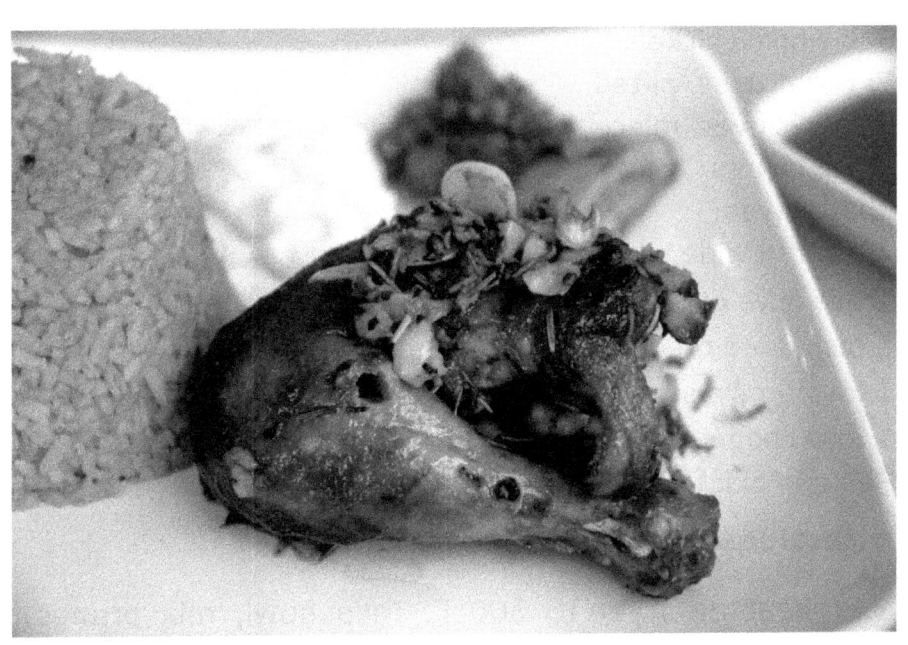

Whole Chicken with Prunes

Cooking Time:

55 minutes

Serve: 4/6

Ingredients:

3 lb whole chicken
½ cup prunes, pitted
3 garlic cloves, minced
2 tbsp capers
2 bay leaves
2 tbsp red wine vinegar
1 tbsp olive oil
1 tbsp dried oregano
1 tbsp brown sugar
1 tbsp chopped parsley
Salt and black pepper to taste

Directions:

1. Preheat air fryer to 360 F. In a bowl, mix prunes, olives, capers, garlic, olive oil, bay leaves, oregano, wine vinegar, salt, and pepper.

2. Spread the mixture on the bottom of a baking dish and place the chicken breast side down on top.

3. Bake for 30 minutes in the fryer, turn it, breast side up, and sprinkle a little bit of brown sugar on top; cook for 10-15 minutes. Let sit for a few minutes before serving.

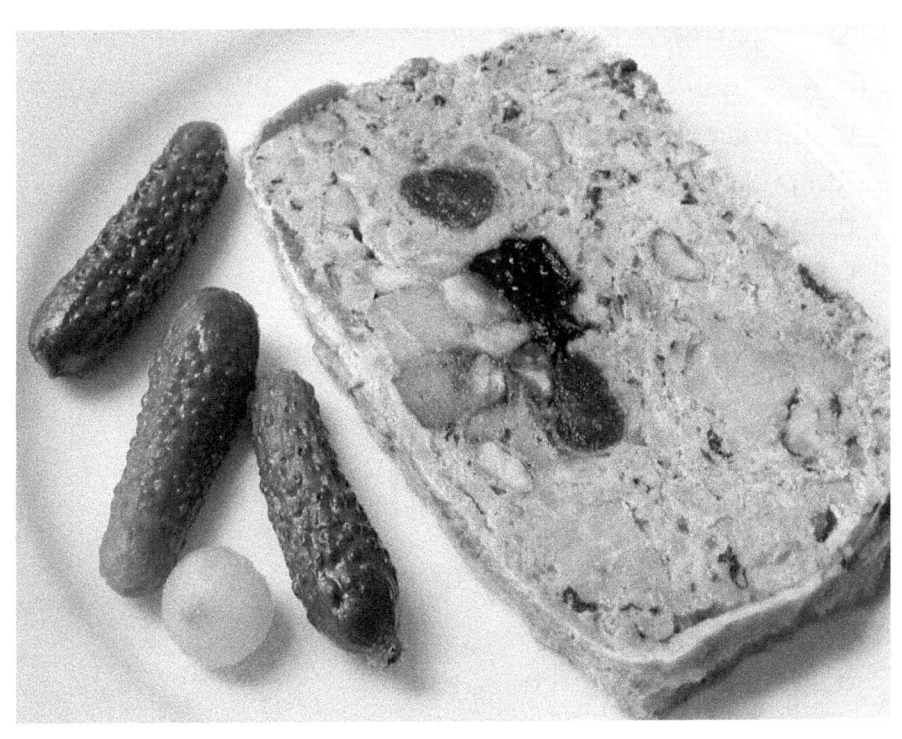

Sticky Chicken Wings with Coleslaw

Cooking Time:

20 minutes

Serve: 2

Ingredients:

10 chicken wings
2 tbsp hot chili sauce
½ tbsp balsamic vinegar
1 tbsp pomegranate molasses
1 tsp brown sugar
1 tsp tomato paste
Salt and black pepper to taste
4 tbsp mayonnaise
½ cup yogurt
1 tbsp lemon juice
½ white cabbage, shredded
1 carrot, grated
1 green onion, sliced
2 tbsp fresh parsley, chopped

Directions:

1. Mix balsamic vinegar, pomegranate molasses, brown sugar, tomato paste, hot chili sauce, salt, and pepper in a bowl.

2. Coat the chicken wings in the mixture, cover, and refrigerate for 30 minutes. In a salad bowl, combine the cabbage, carrot, green onion, and parsley and mix well.

3.In a small bowl, whisk the mayonnaise, yogurt, lemon juice, salt, and pepper. Pour over the coleslaw and mix to combine.

4.Keep in the fridge until ready to use. Preheat air fryer to 350 F. Put the chicken in the air fryer basket and Air Fry for 15 minutes, turning once halfway through. Serve with the chilled coleslaw

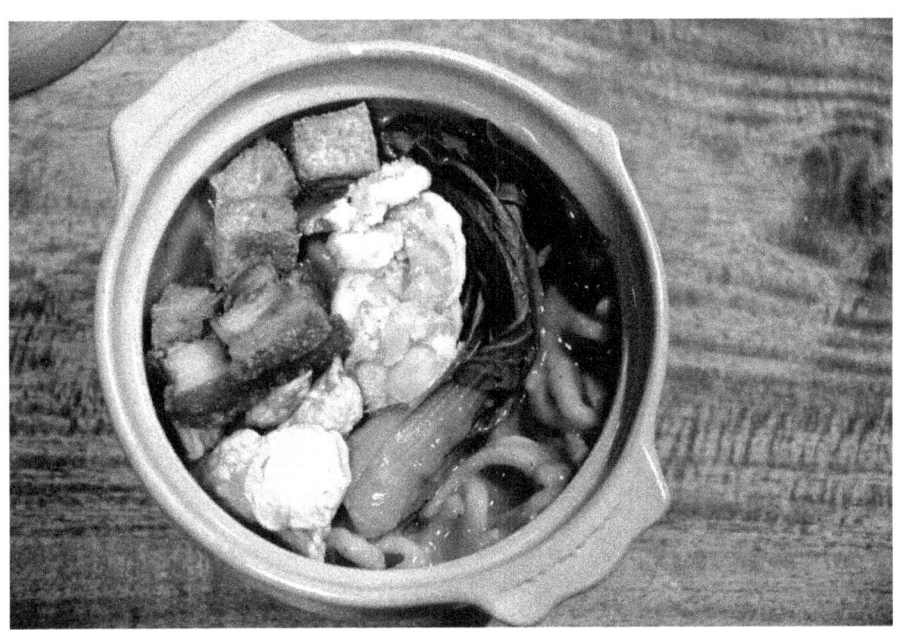

Italian Parmesan Wings with Herbs

Cooking Time:

20 minutes

Serve: 4

Ingredients:

1lb chicken wings
¼ cup butter
¼ cup Parmesan cheese, grated
2 cloves garlic, minced
½ tsp dried oregano
½ tsp dried rosemary
Salt and black pepper to taste
¼ tsp paprika

Directions:

1. Preheat air fryer to 370 F. Place the chicken on a plate and season with salt and pepper.

2. Put in the greased air fryer basket and Air Fry for 7-8 minutes, flipping once. Remove to a greased baking dish.

3. Melt butter in a skillet over medium heat and cook garlic for 1 minute. Stir in paprika, oregano, and rosemary for another minute.

4. Pour the mixture over the chicken, sprinkle with Parmesan cheese, and Bake in the air fryer for 5 minutes. Serve immediately.

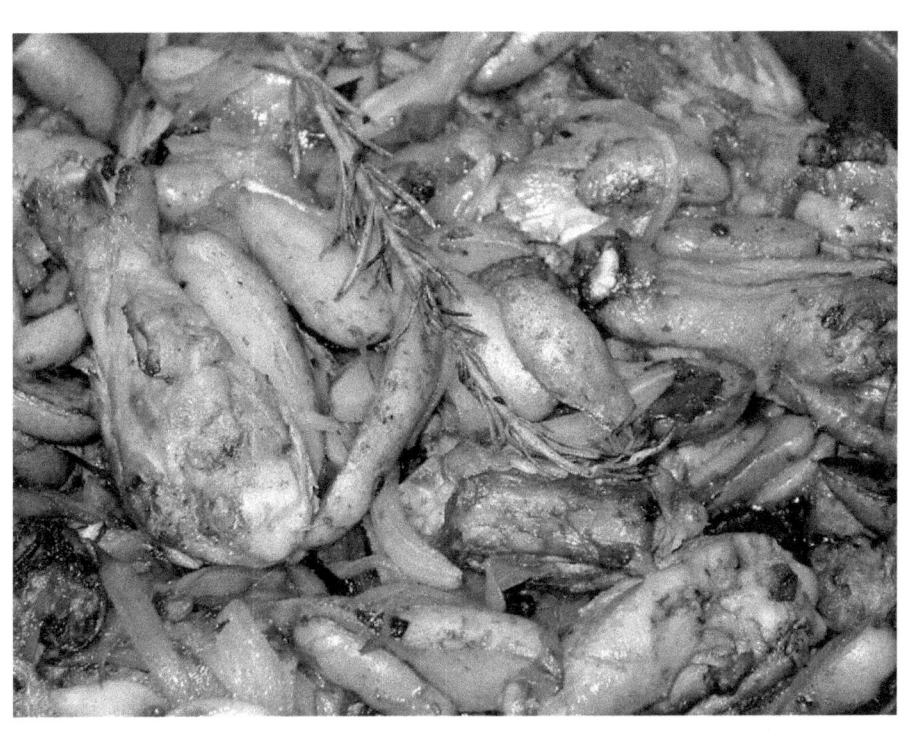

Rice Krispies Chicken Goujons

Cooking Time:

20 minutes

Serve: 4

Ingredients:

1chicken breasts, cut into strips
Salt and black pepper to taste
½ tsp tarragon
½ cup rice Krispies
1 egg, beaten
½ cup plain flour
1 tbsp butter, melted

Directions:

1.Preheat air fryer to 390 F. Line the frying basket with baking paper and grease. Sprinkle the chicken with salt and pepper.

2.Roll the strips in flour, then dip in the egg, and finally coat with rice Krispies.

3.Place the strips in air fryer, drizzle with melted butter, and Air Fry for 12-14 minutes, shaking once. Serve hot.

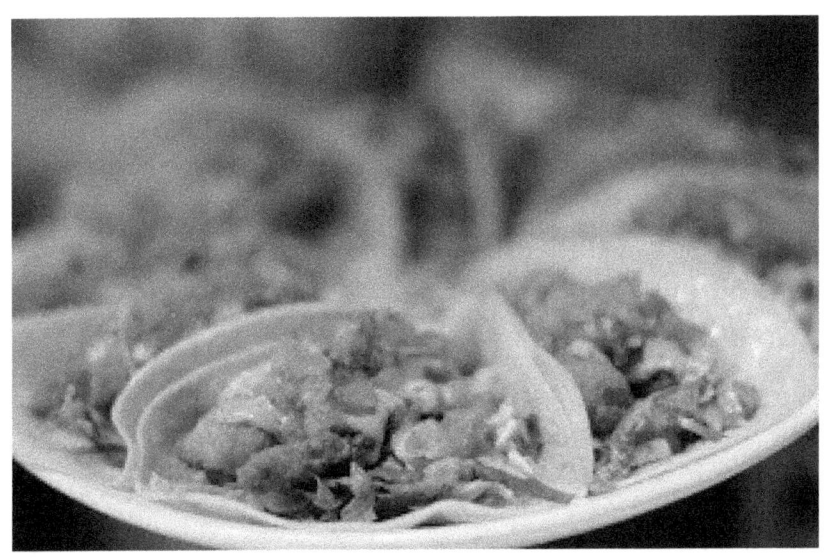

Crispy Chicken Tenders with Hot Aioli

Cooking Time:

20 minutes

Serve: 4

Ingredients:

1 lb chicken breasts, cut into strips
4 tbsp olive oil
1 cup breadcrumbs
Salt and black pepper to taste
½ tbsp garlic powder
½ tbsp cayenne pepper
½ cup mayonnaise
2 tbsp lemon juice
½ tbsp ground chili

DIRECTIONS

1. Preheat air fryer to 390 F. Mix breadcrumbs, salt, pepper, garlic powder, and cayenne pepper and spread onto a plate.

2. Brush the chicken strips with some olive oil. Roll them in the breadcrumb mixture until well coated.

3. Arrange the strips on a greased air fryer basket in an even layer and Bake for 12 minutes, turning once halfway through.

4.To prepare the hot aioli: place the mayo with the lemon juice and ground chili in a small bowl and whisk to combine well. Serve with the chicken tenders and enjoy!

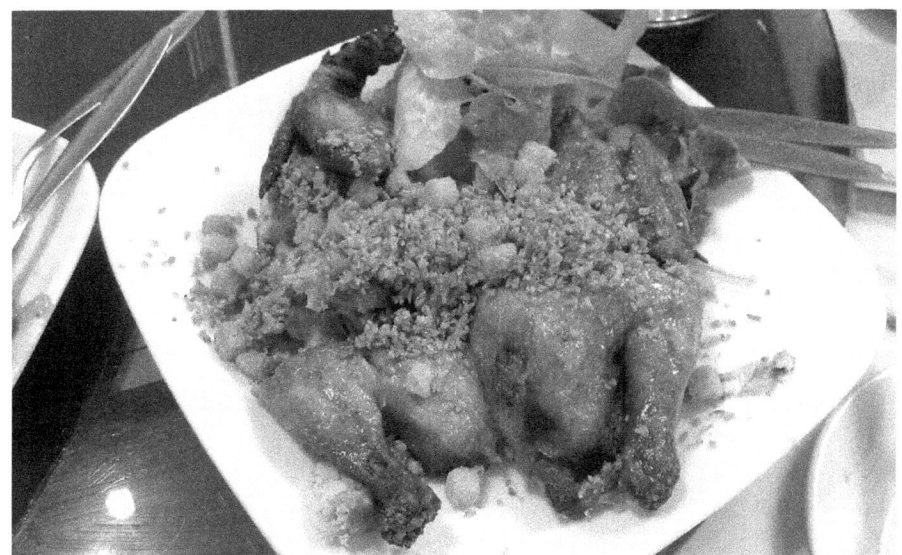

Jerusalem Matzah & Chicken Schnitzels

Cooking Time:

10 minutes

Serve: 4

Ingredients:

4 chicken breasts
1 cup panko breadcrumbs
2 tbsp Parmesan cheese, grated
6 sage leaves, chopped
½ cup fine matzah meal
2 beaten eggs

Directions:

1. Pound the chicken to ¼-inch thickness using a rolling pin.

2. In a bowl, add Parmesan cheese, sage, and breadcrumbs.

3. Toss chicken with matzah meal, dip in eggs, then coat well with bread crumbs.

4. Preheat air fryer to 390 F. Spray both sides of chicken breasts with cooking spray and Air Fry in the frying basket for 14-16 minutes, turning once halfway through until golden. Serve warm.

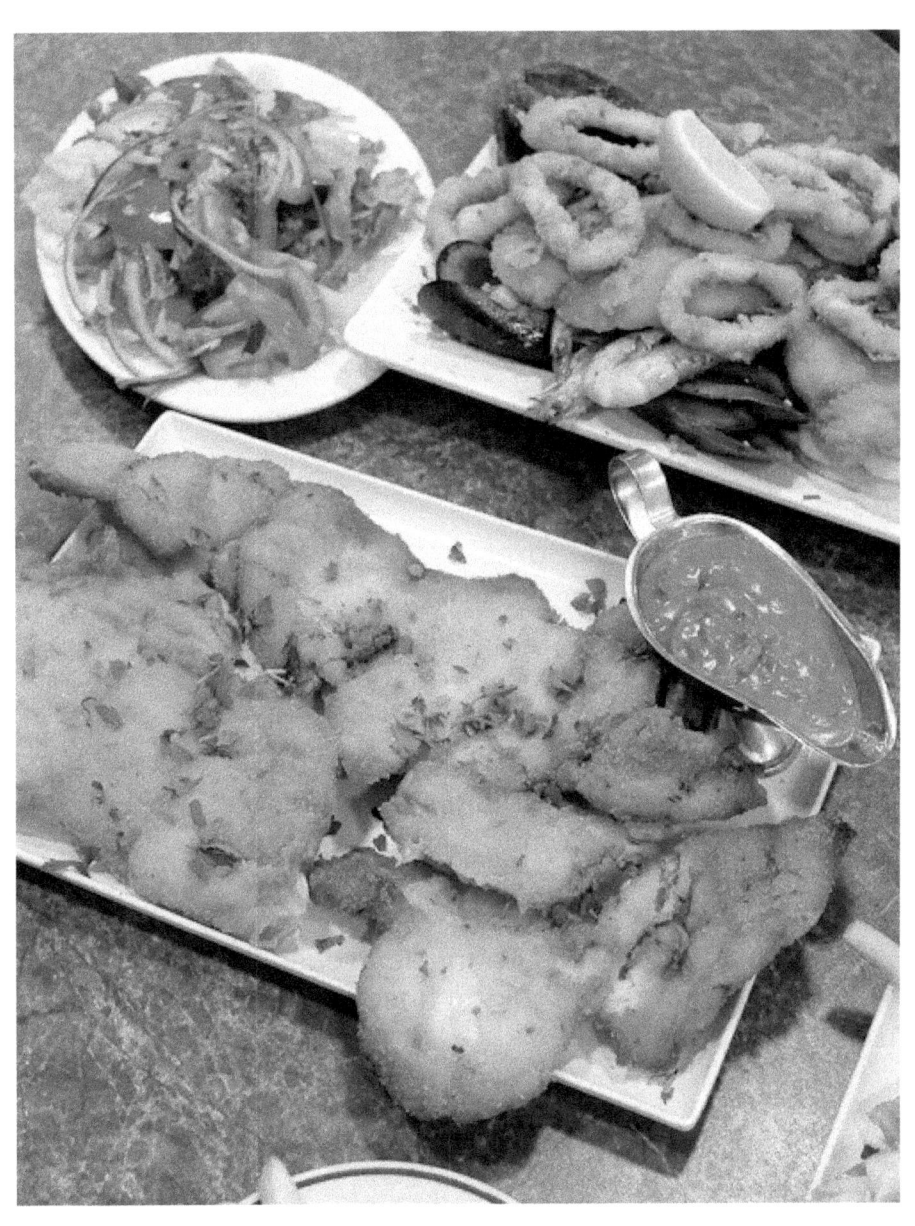

Creamy Asiago Chicken

Cooking Time:

25 minutes

Serve: 4

Ingredients:

4 chicken breasts, cubed
½ tsp garlic powder
1 cup mayonnaise
½ cup Asiago cheese, grated
Salt and black pepper to taste
2 tbsp fresh basil, chopped

Directions:

1. Preheat air fryer to 380 F. In a bowl, mix Asiago cheese, mayonnaise, garlic powder, and salt. Add in the chicken and toss to coat.

2. Place the coated chicken in the greased frying basket. Bake for 15 minutes, shaking once. Serve sprinkled with freshly chopped basil.

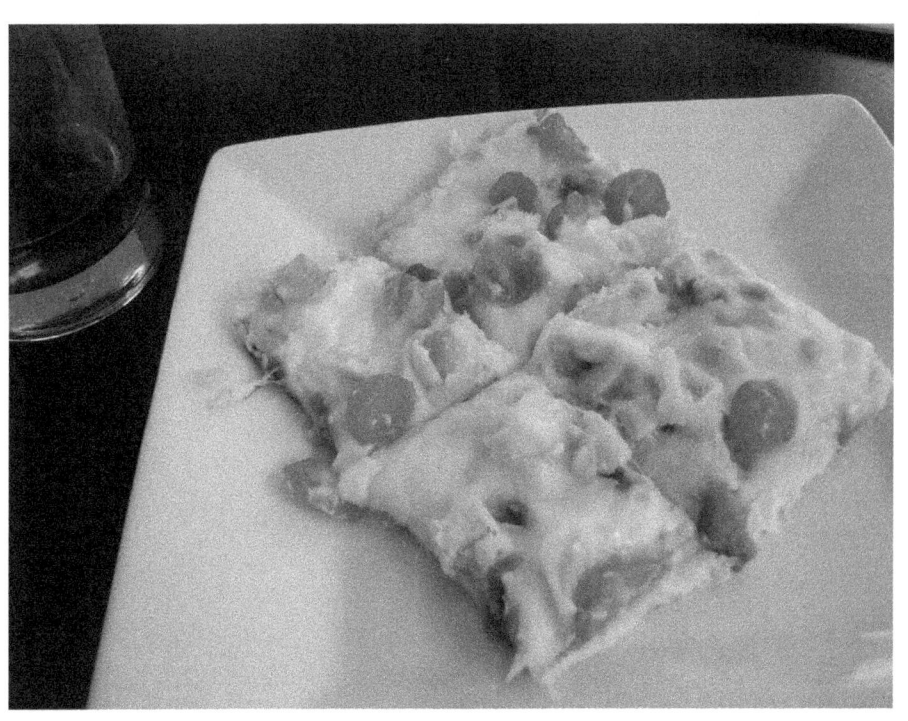

Creamy Onion Chicken

Cooking Time:

30 minutes

Serve: 4

Ingredients:

4 chicken breasts, cubed 1 ½ cups onion soup mix 1 cup mushroom soup ½ cup heavy cream

Directions:

1. Preheat air fryer to 400 F. Warm mushroom soup, onion mix, and heavy cream in a frying pan over low heat for 1 minute.

2. Pour the mixture over the chicken and let sit for 25 minutes. Transfer the chicken to the air fryer and Bake for 15 minutes, shaking once. Serve topped with the remaining sauce.

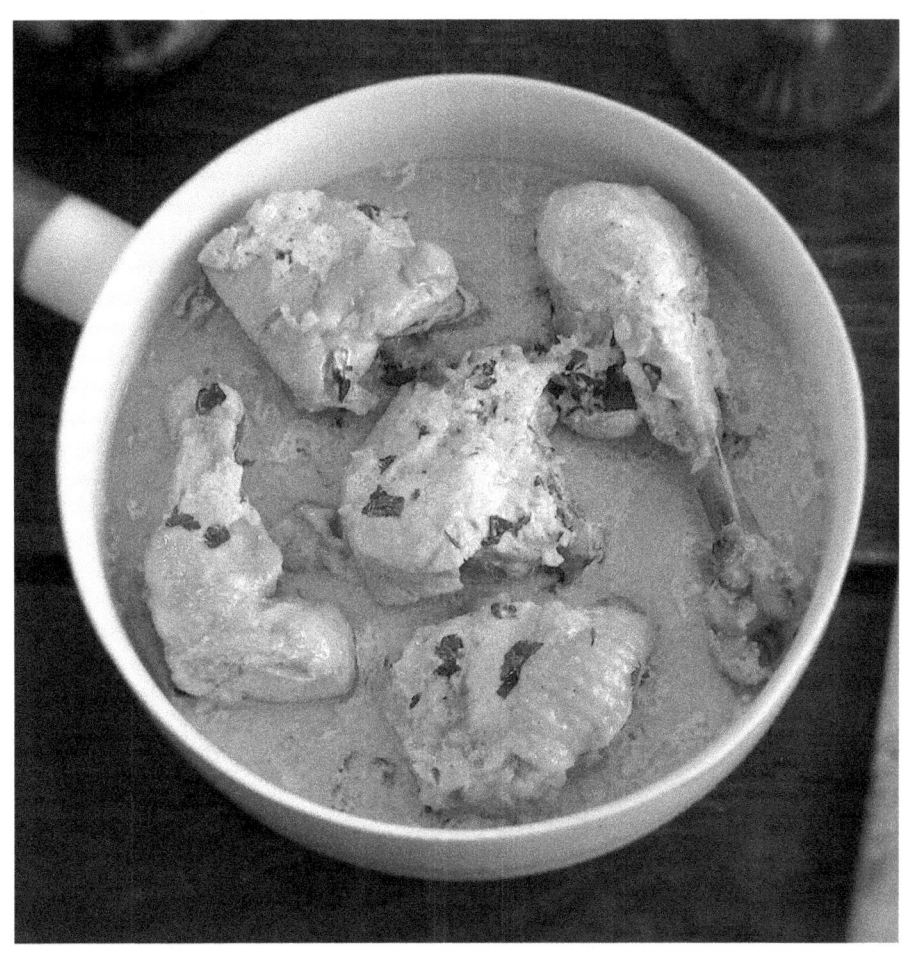

Cauli-Oat Crusted Drumsticks

Cooking Time:

25 minutes

Serve: 4

Ingredients:

8 chicken drumsticks
½ tsp dried oregano
½ tsp dried thyme
2 oz oats
10 oz cauliflower florets, steamed
1 egg
1 tsp ground cayenne pepper
Salt and black pepper to taste

Directions:

1. Preheat air fryer to 350 F. Rub the drumsticks with salt and pepper.

2. Place all remaining ingredients, except for the egg, in a food processor.

3. Process until smooth. Dip each drumstick in the egg first and then in the oat mixture. Arrange them on the frying basket and Air Fry for 14-16 minutes, flipping once.

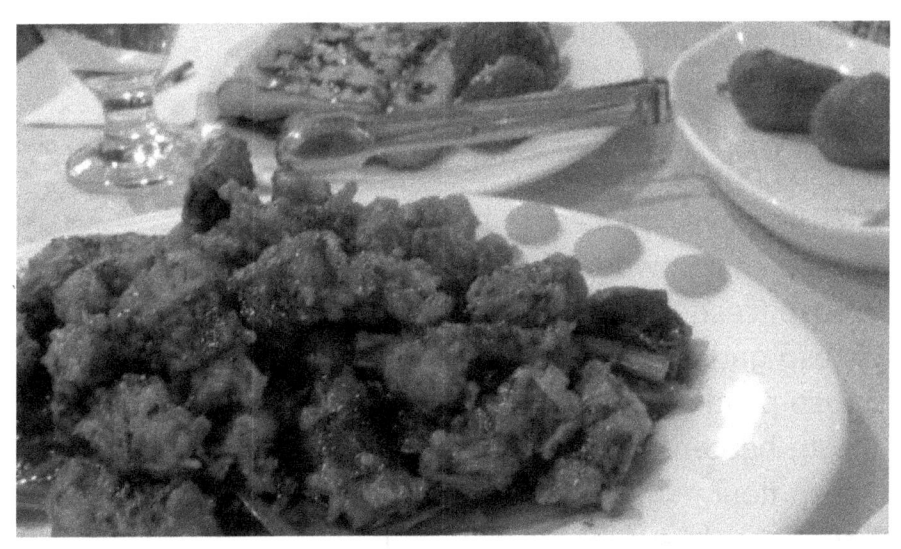

Chicken Asian Lollipop

Cooking Time:

30 minutes

Serve: 4

Ingredients:

1lb mini chicken drumsticks
½ tbsp soy sauce
1 tbsp lime juice
Salt and black pepper to taste
1 tbsp cornstarch
1 garlic clove, minced
½ tbsp chili powder
½ tbsp fresh cilantro, chopped
½ tbsp garlic-ginger paste
1 tbsp plain vinegar
1 egg, beaten
1 tbsp flour
1 tbsp maple syrup

Directions:

1. Mix garlic-ginger paste, chili powder, maple syrup, soy sauce, cilantro, vinegar, egg, garlic, and salt in a bowl.

2. Add the chicken and toss to coat. Stir in cornstarch, flour, and lime juice. Preheat air fryer to 350 F. Place the drumsticks in the greased frying basket and Air Fry for 5-7 minutes.

3.Turn and continue cooking for 5 more minutes. Remove to a serving platter and serve with tomato dip.

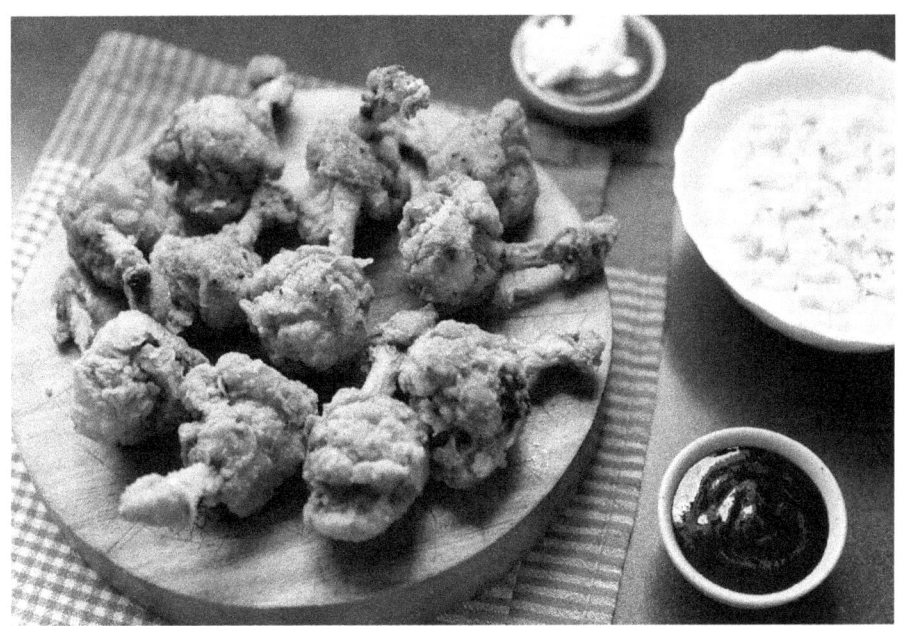

Moroccan Turkey Meatballs

Cooking Time:

30 minutes

Serve: 4

Ingredients:

½ cup couscous
1 cucumber, chopped
1 egg, beaten
1 lb ground turkey
2 garlic cloves, minced
½ cup panko bread crumbs
1 tbsp soy sauce
¼ cup + 1 tbsp hoisin sauce
1 tsp sriracha sauce
Salt and black pepper to taste

Directions:

1.In a bowl, mix couscous and 1 cup of boiling water. Cover and let sit for 8-10 minutes. Fluff with a fork.

2.Preheat air fryer to 360 F. Mix the turkey, panko breadcrumbs, egg, soy sauce, 1 tablespoon of hoisin sauce, garlic, salt, and black pepper in a bowl. Make small balls with a tablespoon.

3.Combine the remaining hoisin sauce and sriracha in a small bowl to make a glaze and set aside.

4.Put the meatballs in the greased fryer basket in a single later and air fry for 8 minutes.

5.Generously brush the meatballs with the glaze and cook 4-7 more minutes until cooked through.

6.Season the couscous with salt and mix with the cucumber. Top with the meatballs and serve.

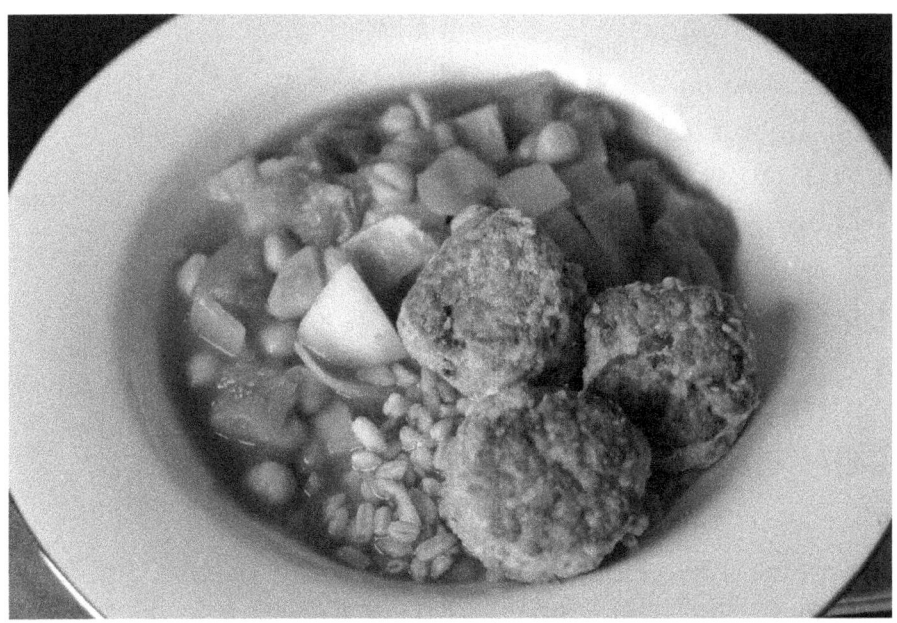

Roasted Turkey with Brussels Sprouts

Cooking Time:

60 minutes

Serve: 6

Ingredients:

1lb turkey breast
2 garlic cloves, minced
1 tbsp olive oil
2 tsp Dijon mustard
1 ½ tsp rosemary
1 lb Brussels sprouts, halved
Salt and black pepper to taste

Directions:

1. Preheat your Air Fryer to 375°F. Mix the garlic, olive oil, Dijon mustard, rosemary, sage, thyme, salt, and pepper in a bowl and make a paste.

2. Smear the paste all over the turkey breast. Put the turkey breast in the greased fryer basket and air fry for 20 minutes.

3. Turn it over and baste it with any drippings from the bottom drawer. Add in the Brussels sprouts and air fry for 20 more minutes. Let the turkey sit for 10 minutes before slicing. Serve with Brussels sprouts.

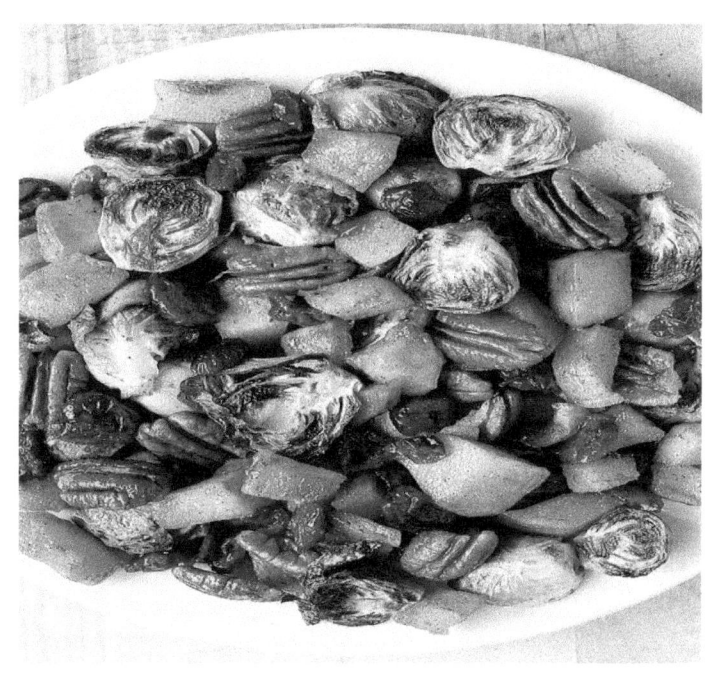

Greek-Style Chicken Wings

Cooking Time:

25 minutes

Serve: 4

Directions:

1 lb chicken wings
1 tbsp fresh parsley, chopped
Salt and black pepper to taste
1 tbsp cashew butter
1 garlic clove, minced
1 tbsp yogurt
1 tsp honey
½ tbsp vinegar
½ tbsp garlic chili sauce

Directions:

1. Preheat air fryer to 360 F. Season the wings with salt and pepper and Air Fry in the greased frying basket for 15 minutes, shaking once.

2. In a bowl, mix the remaining ingredients. Transfer the wings to a greased baking dish, top with sauce, and cook in the air fryer basket for 5 minutes. Serve warm.

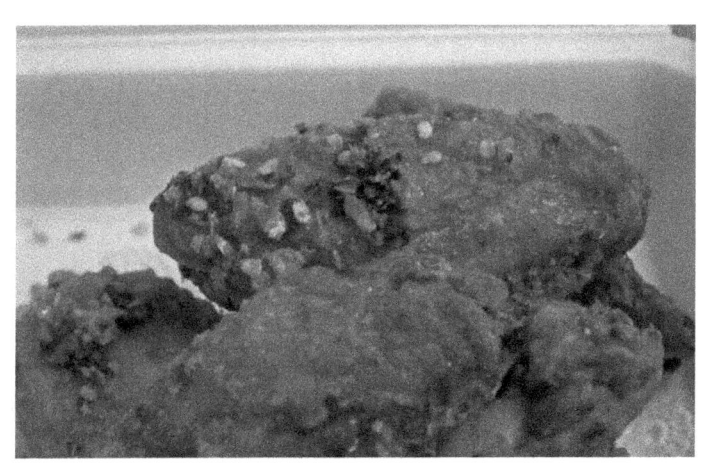

Chicken & Jalapeño Quesadilla

Cooking Time:

20 minutes

Serve: 4

Ingredients:

8 tortillas
2 cups Monterey Jack cheese, shredded
½ cup cooked chicken, shredded
1 cup canned fire-roasted jalapeño peppers, chopped
1 beaten egg, to seal tortillas

Directions:

1. Preheat air fryer to 390 F. Divide chicken, cheese, and jalapeño peppers between 4 tortillas. Seal the tortillas with beaten egg.

2. Grease with cooking spray. In batches, place in the air fryer basket and Bake for 12 minutes, turning once halfway through. Serve with green salsa.

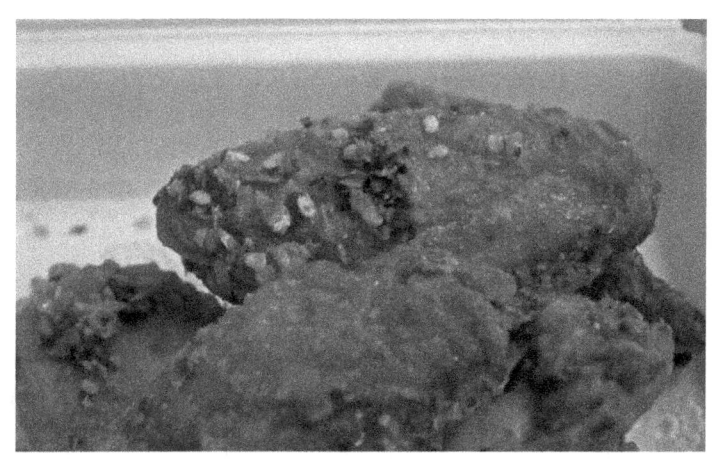

Chicken & Jalapeño Quesadilla

Cooking Time:

20 minutes

Serve: 4

Ingredients:

8 tortillas
2 cups Monterey Jack cheese, shredded
½ cup cooked chicken, shredded
1 cup canned fire-roasted jalapeño peppers, chopped
1 beaten egg, to seal tortillas

Directions:

1. Preheat air fryer to 390 F. Divide chicken, cheese, and jalapeño peppers between 4 tortillas. Seal the tortillas with beaten egg.

2. Grease with cooking spray. In batches, place in the air fryer basket and Bake for 12 minutes, turning once halfway through. Serve with green salsa.

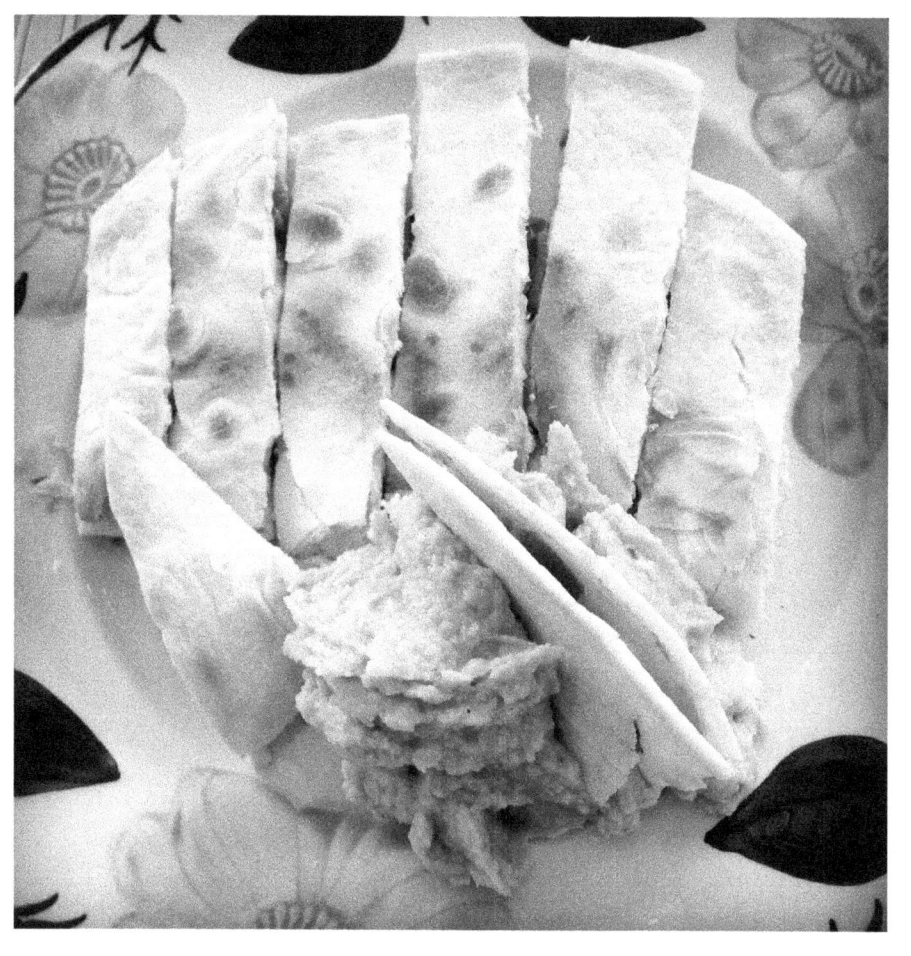

Chicken Fingers with Red Mayo Dip

Cooking Time:

35 minutes

Serve: 4

Ingredients:

1 lb chicken breasts, cut into finger-sized strips
1 tbsp olive oil
½ tsp paprika
½ tsp garlic powder
½ cup seasoned bread crumbs
1 tsp dried parsley
Salt and black pepper to taste
½ cup mayonnaise
2 tbsp ketchup
½ tsp garlic powder
½ tsp sweet chili sauce

Directions:

1. Preheat air fryer to 375 F. Toss the chicken with salt, pepper, paprika, and garlic powder in a bowl, coating the chicken evenly.

2. Add olive oil and toss again. Mix the breadcrumbs and parsley in a shallow bowl and coat each piece of chicken. Put the chicken in a single layer in the greased basket.

3. Air Fry for 10 minutes. Turn the chicken over, spray with olive oil again, and cook for 8-10 more minutes

until golden and crisp.

4.In a bowl, whisk the mayonnaise, ketchup, garlic powder, chili sauce, salt, and pepper. Pour the dip into a serving bowl and serve with the chicken fingers. Enjoy!

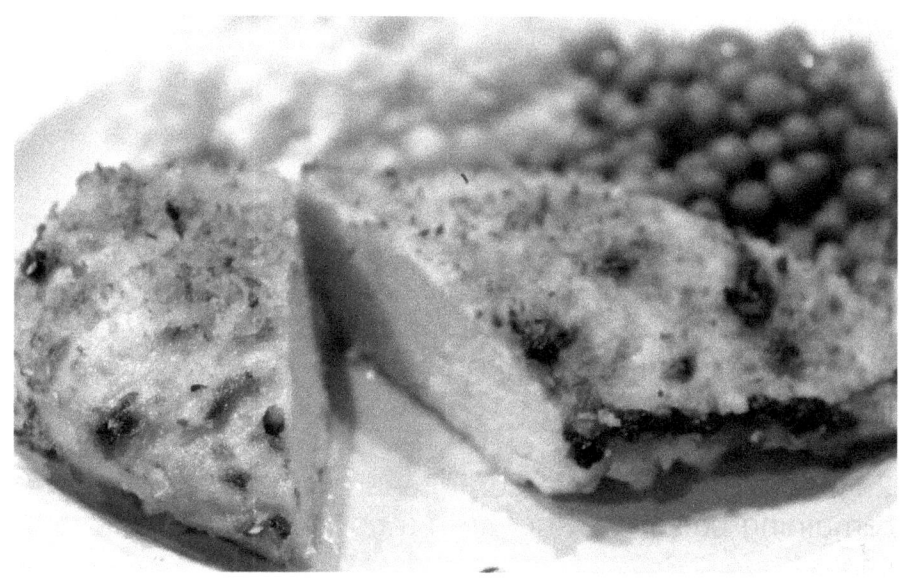

Balsamic Chicken with Green Beans

Cooking Time:

40 minutes

Serve: 4

Ingredients:

1 lb chicken breasts, sliced
1 lb green beans, trimmed
¾ cup balsamic vinegar
2 tbsp olive oil
1 lb cherry tomatoes, halved
1 garlic clove, minced

Directions:

1. In a bowl, add ½ cup of balsamic vinegar and chicken and stir to coat. Refrigerate for at least 1 hour. Preheat air fryer to 375 F.

2. Mix the green beans, garlic, cherry tomatoes, and the remaining balsamic vinegar in a bowl and toss until well coated.

3. Put the veggies in the greased fryer basket and air fry for 8 minutes. Shake the basket and fry for 5-7 more minutes until the beans are crisp and tender and the tomatoes are soft and slightly charred.

4. Remove and cover with foil to keep warm. Spray the fryer basket with olive oil. Put the chicken in a single layer in the fryer basket and air fry for 7 minutes.

5.Flip the chicken and cook for 5-8 more minutes. Serve the chicken with the veggies.

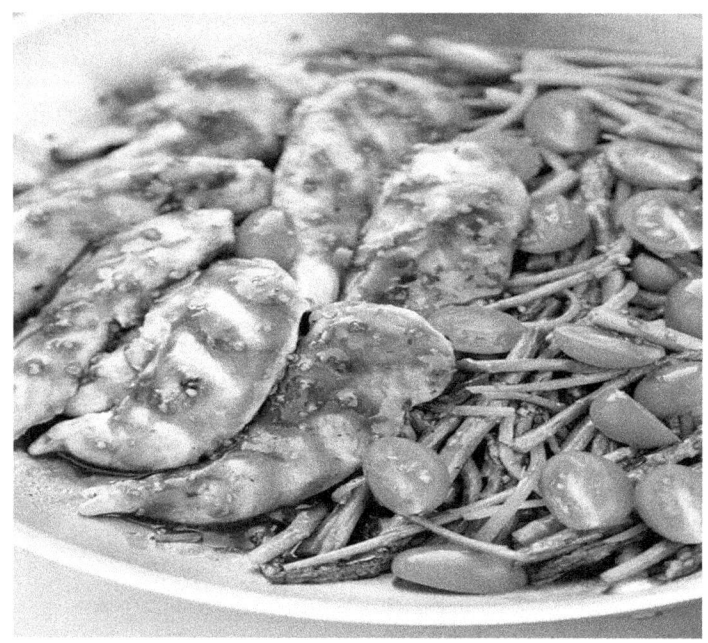

Chicken Teriyaki

Cooking Time:

20 minutes

Serve: 4

Ingredients:

1 lb chicken tenderloins
⅓ cup soy sauce
⅓ cup honey
3 tbsp white vinegar
1 ½ tsp dried thyme
½ tsp cayenne pepper
½ tsp ground allspice
2 cups cooked brown rice
2 cups steamed broccoli florets
1 tsp ground black pepper
1 tbsp fresh cilantro, chopped
2 green onions, chopped

Directions:

1. Mix soy sauce, honey, white vinegar, thyme, black pepper, cayenne pepper, and allspice in a bowl to make a marinade.

2. Toss the tenderloins in the marinade to coat. Cover and refrigerate for 30 minutes.

3. Preheat air fryer to 380 F. Remove the chicken the marinade; keep the marinade for later.

4.Put the chicken in a single layer in the greased fryer basket and air fry for 6 minutes. Turn the chicken and brush with the remaining marinade. Cook for 5- 7 more minutes.

5.Divide the brown rice, steamed broccoli, and chicken tenderloins between 4 bowls. Top with cilantro and green onions and serve immediately.

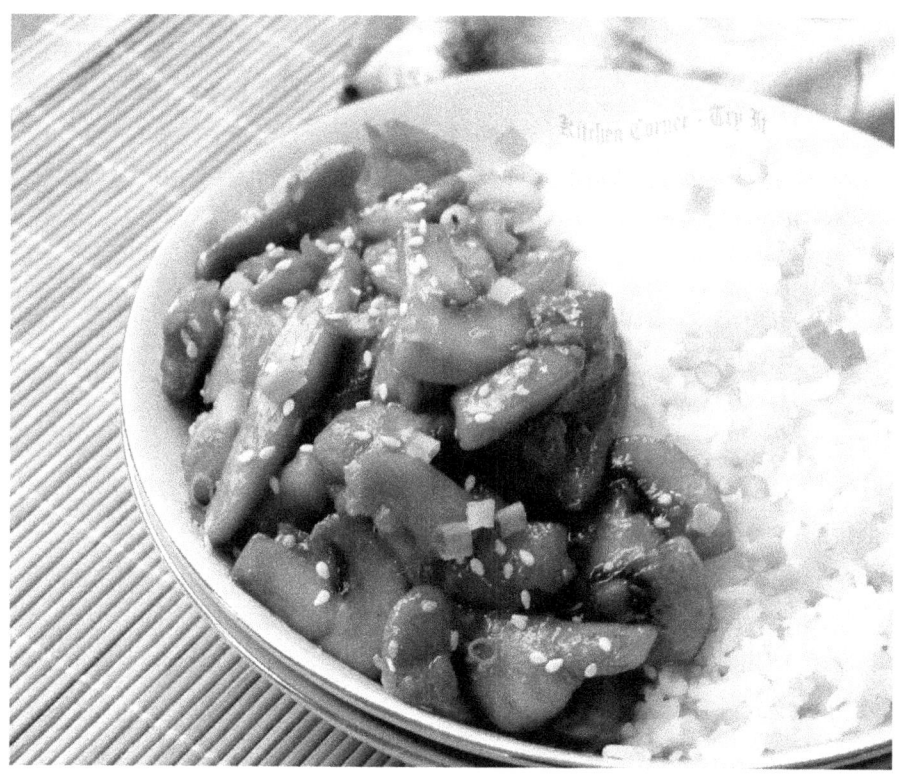

Spinach Loaded Chicken Breasts

Cook Time:

15 minutes

Servings: 4

Ingredients:

1 cup spinach, chopped

4 tbsp cottage cheese, crumbled

2 chicken breasts Juice of ½ lime

2 tbsp Italian seasoning

2 tbsp olive oil

Directions:

1. Preheat air fryer to 390 F. Grease the basket with cooking spray.

2. Mix spinach and cottage cheese in a bowl. Halve the breasts with a knife and flatten them with a meat mallet. Season with Italian seasoning.

3. Divide the spinach/cheese mixture between the chicken pieces.

4. Roll up to form cylinders and use toothpicks to secure them. Brush with olive oil and place them in the frying basket.

5. Bake for 7-8 minutes, flip, and cook for 6 minutes. Serve warm.

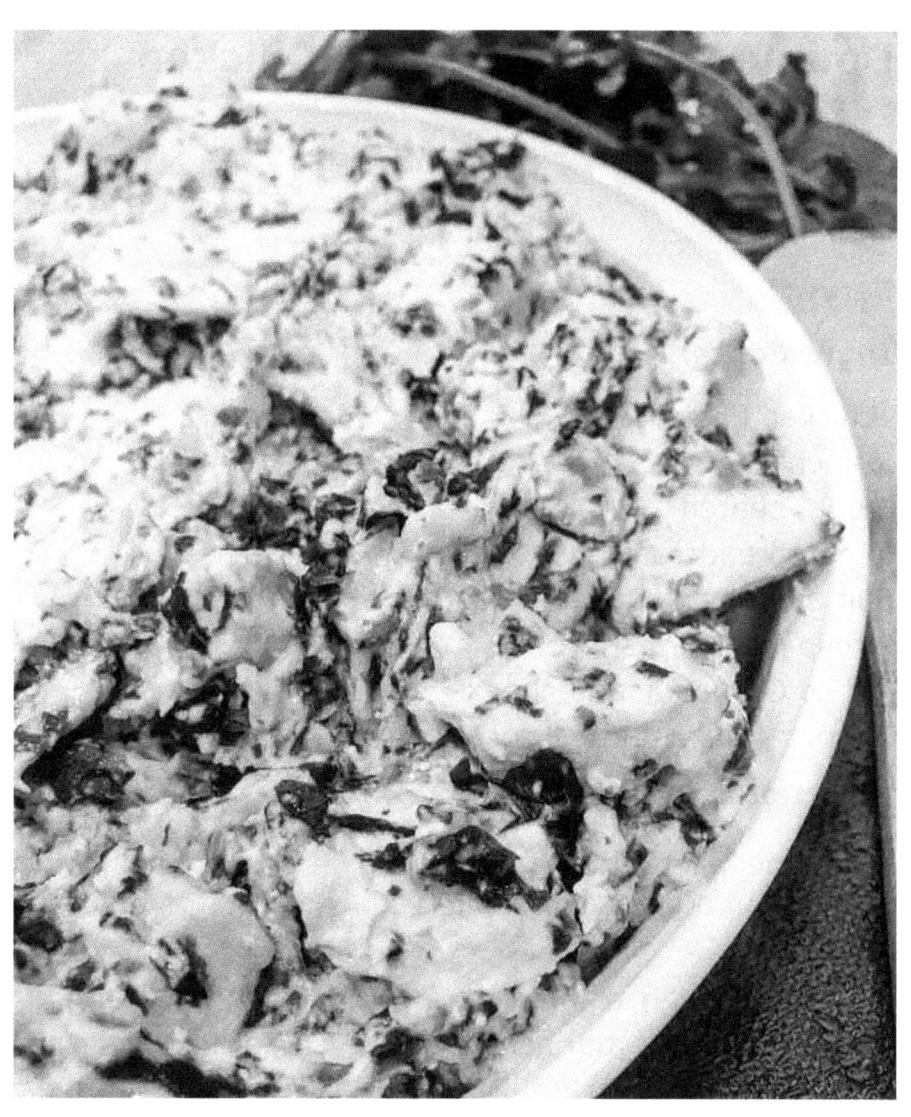

Double Cheese Marinara Chicken

Cooking Time:

15 minutes

Serve: 2

Ingredients:

1 chicken fillets,
½-inch thick
1 egg, beaten
½ cup breadcrumbs
Salt and black pepper to taste
2 tbsp marinara sauce
2 tbsp Grana Padano cheese, grated
2 mozzarella cheese slices

Directions:

1. Dip the fillets in the egg, then in the crumbs, and arrange on a greased baking dish.

2. Air Fry in the frying basket for 7-8 minutes at 400 F. Turn, top with marinara sauce, Grana Padano and mozzarella cheeses, and bake further for 5-6 more minutes. Serve warm.

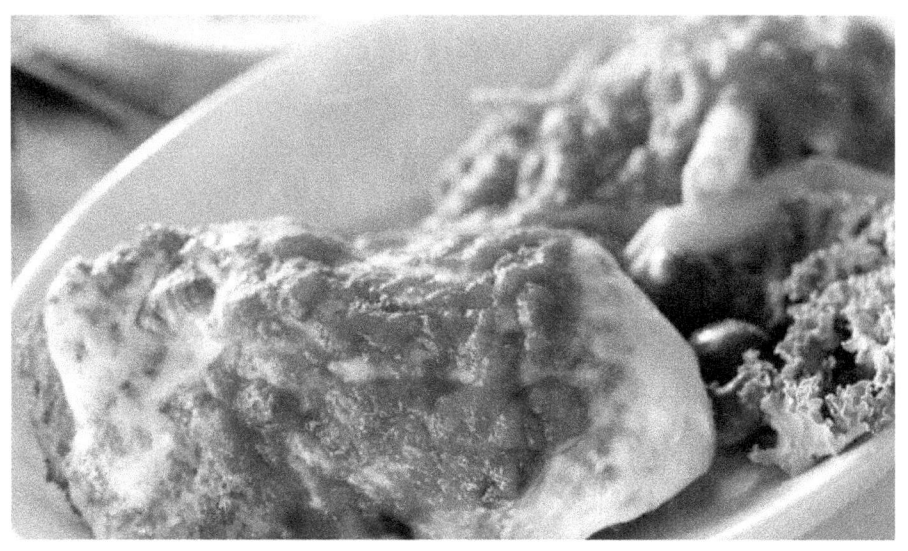

Chicken Thighs with Marinara Sauce

Cooking Time:

15 minutes

Serve: 4

Ingredients:

½ cup panko breadcrumbs
2 tbsp Parmesan cheese, grated
Salt and black pepper to taste
1 tbsp olive oil
1 tsp Italian seasoning
4 chicken thighs
½ cup spicy marinara sauce
½ cup mozzarella cheese

Directions:

1. Preheat air fryer to 350 F. In a bowl, combine breadcrumbs, Italian seasoning, and Parmesan cheese.

2. Coat the chicken with olive oil, salt, and pepper. Dip in the breadcrumb/cheese mixture; shake off any excess.

3. Place the thighs in the greased fryer and Air Fry for 6-8 minutes. Slide the basket out and top with marinara sauce and mozzarella cheese. Slide back in, and cook for another 4-5 minutes. Serve.

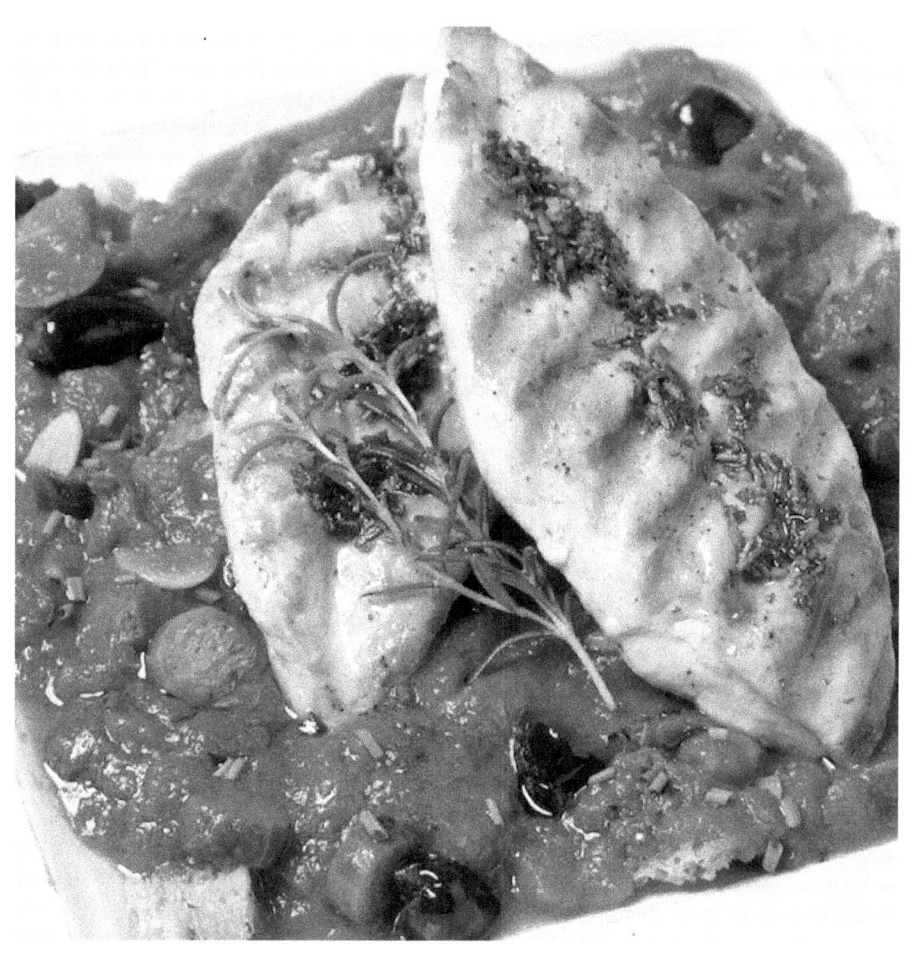

Whole Roasted Chicken

Cooking Time:

65 minutes

Serve: 4

Ingredients:

3.5-ounce whole chicken
2 tbsp olive oil
1 tsp garlic powder
1 tsp paprika
½ tsp oregano
Salt and black pepper to taste
1 lemon, cut into quarters
5 garlic cloves

Directions:

1. In a bowl, combine olive oil, garlic powder, paprika, oregano, salt, and pepper, and mix well to make a paste.

2. Rub the chicken with the paste and stuff lemon and garlic cloves into the cavity. Place the chicken in the air fryer, breast side down, and tuck the legs and wings tips under.

3. Bake for 45 minutes at 360 F. Flip the chicken to breast side up and cook for another 15-20 minutes. Let rest for 5-6 minutes, then carve, and serve.

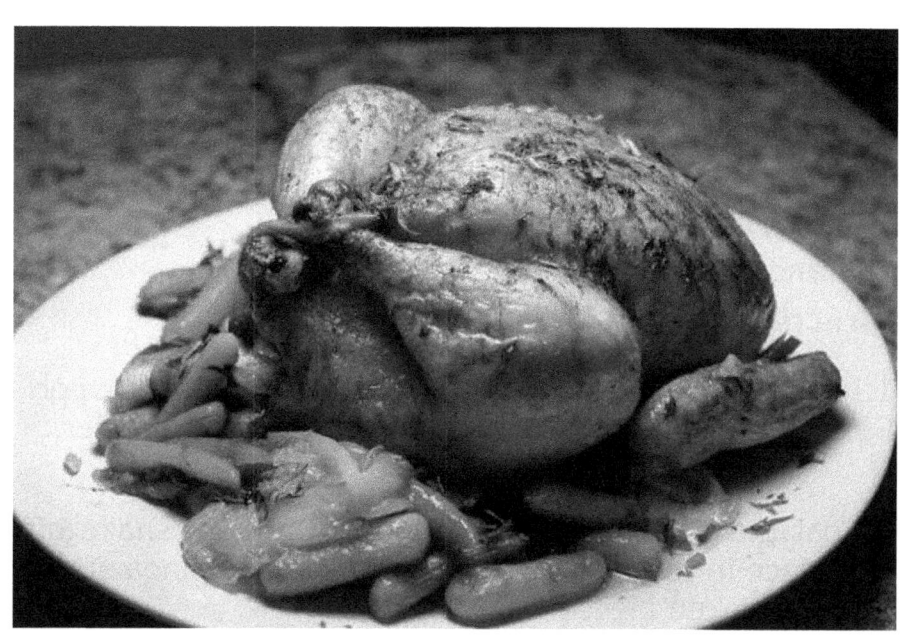

Quinoa Chicken Nuggets

Cooking Time:

15 minutes

Serve: 4

Ingredients:

1 chicken breasts, cut into bite-size chunks
½ cup cooked quinoa, cooled
½ cup flour
1 egg
½ tsp cayenne pepper
Salt and black pepper to taste

Directions:

1. In a bowl, beat the egg with salt and black pepper. Spread flour on a plate and mix with cayenne pepper.

2. Coat the chicken in flour, then in the egg, shake off and place in the quinoa. Press firmly such quinoa sticks on the chicken pieces.

3. Spray with cooking spray and Air Fry the nuggets in the greased frying basket for 14-16 minutes at 360 F, turning once halfway through. Serve hot.

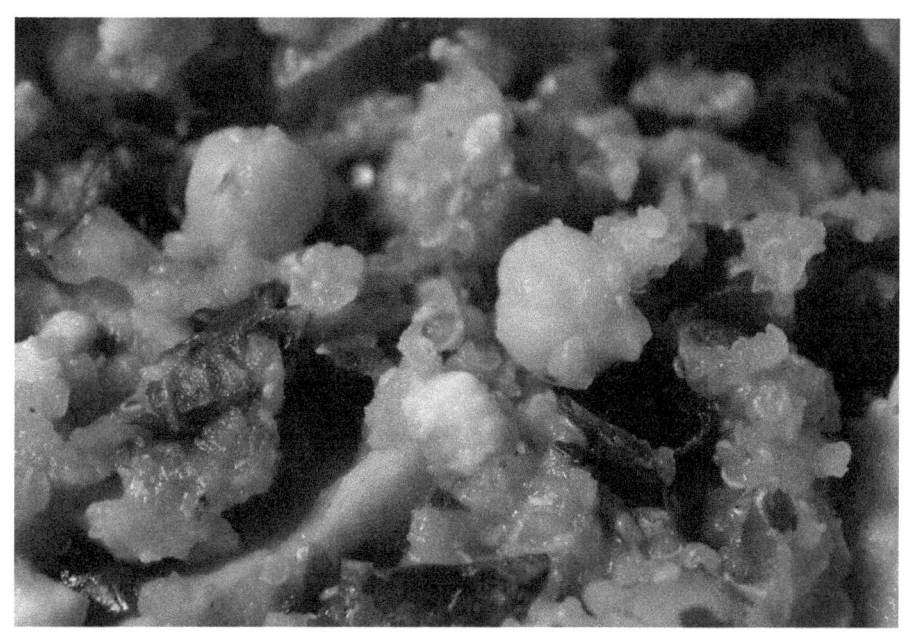

Tex-Mex Seasoned Chicken

Cooking Time:

25 minutes

Serve: 4

Ingredients:

1 mixed bell peppers, cut into chunks
1 red onion, sliced
1 lb chicken tenderloins, cut into strips
1 tbsp olive oil
2 tbsp cilantro, chopped
1 tbsp taco seasoning

Directions:

1. Preheat air fryer to 375 F. Mix the chicken, bell peppers, onion, 1 tbsp olive oil, and fajita seasoning mix in a large bowl and stir until the chicken is coated.

2. Put the chicken and veggies in the greased fryer basket and spray with olive oil.

3. Air fry for 7 minutes, shake the basket, and cook for 5-8 minutes, making sure the chicken is thoroughly cooked, and the veggies are starting to char. Serve topped with cilantro.

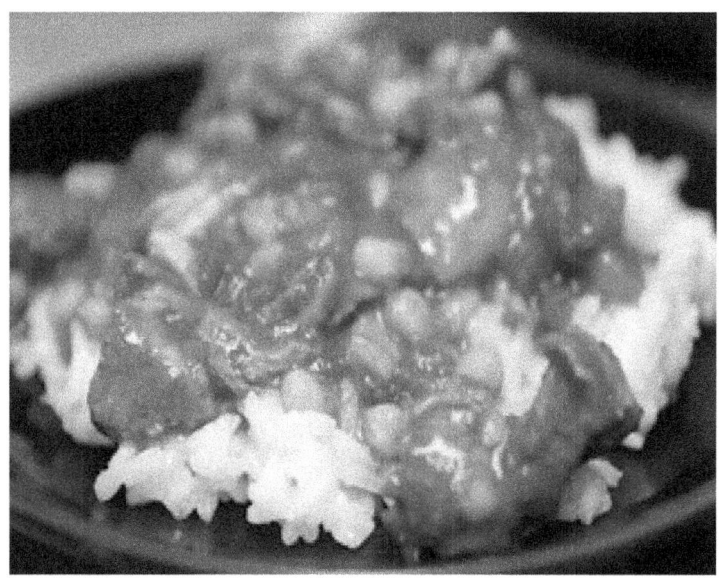

Cajun Chicken Tenders

Cooking Time:

25 minutes

Serve: 4

Ingredients:

1 lb chicken breasts, sliced
3 eggs
1 cup flour
2 tbsp olive oil
½ tbsp garlic powder
1 tbsp salt
1 tbsp Cajun seasoning
¼ cup milk

Directions:

1. Season the chicken with salt, black pepper, garlic powder, and Cajun seasoning. Pour the flour on a plate. In another bowl, whisk the eggs, milk, and olive oil.

2. Preheat air fryer to 370 F. Line a baking sheet with parchment paper. Dip the chicken into the egg mixture, and then in the

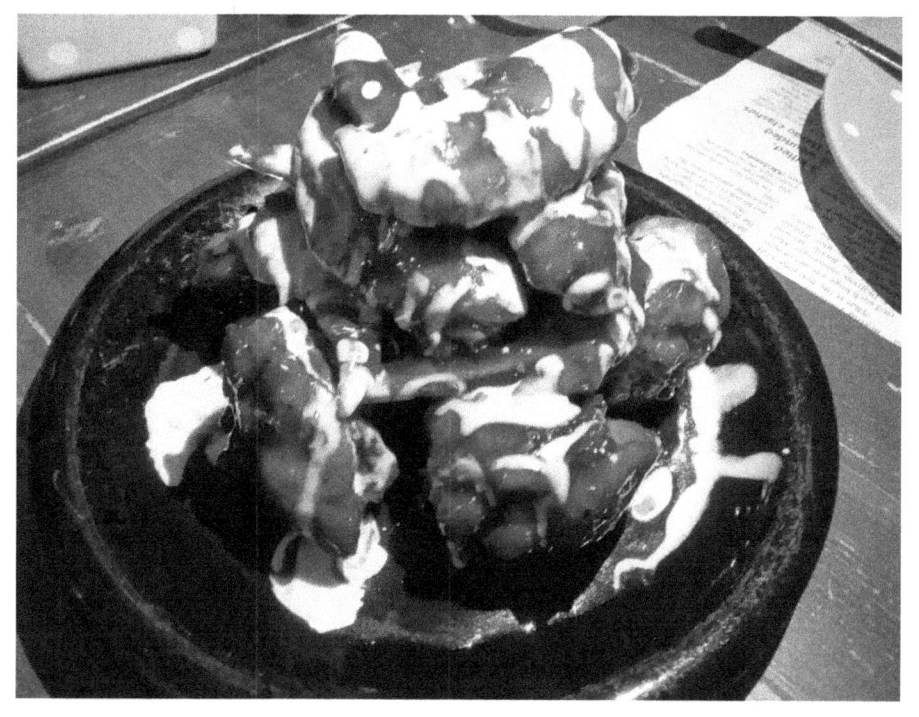

www.ingramcontent.com/pod-product-compliance
Lightning Source LLC
Chambersburg PA
CBHW070723030426
42336CB00013B/1909